Medical Genetics and Genomics

Medical Genetics and Genomics

Questions for Board Review

Benjamin D. Solomon, MD

Pediatrician and Clinical Geneticist

WILEY Blackwell

Registered Offices
John Wiley & Sons, Inc., 111 River Street, Hoboken, NJ 07030, USA
John Wiley & Sons Ltd, The Atrium, Southern Gate, Chichester, West Sussex, PO19 8SQ, UK

Editorial Office
9600 Garsington Road, Oxford, OX4 2DQ, UK

For details of our global editorial offices, customer services, and more information about Wiley products visit us at www. wiley.com.

Wiley also publishes its books in a variety of electronic formats and by print-on-demand. Some content that appears in standard print versions of this book may not be available in other formats.

Library of Congress Cataloging-in-Publication Data applied for
Paperback ISBN: 9781119847182

Cover Design: Wiley
Cover Image: © sorbetto/Getty Images

Set in 10/12pt WarnockPro by Straive, Pondicherry, India

Printed in Singapore
M119322_290722

Dedication

For my family, who loves genetics.

Contents

Introduction

I hope that this book may be of use to many genetics and other medical trainees, including those in various genetics/genomics-based residencies, fellowships, and genetic counseling training programs. I anticipate that others, such as medical students, clinicians, or laboratorians who may encounter patients with known or suspected genetic conditions, may also benefit. These questions can be used to study for board or other standardized examinations. Trainees may also want to use these questions to brush up before a genetics or related rotation. As genetics and genomics extends into more and more areas of medicine, this knowledge is increasingly relevant to just about every field of medicine, including cardiology, gastroenterology, immunology, neonatology, nephrology, neurology, oncology, ophthalmology, pathology, and rheumatology, to name just a handful.

I also want to briefly mention a few points about the questions assembled here.

First, based on polling colleagues and trainees, I decided to break up the questions into different thematic areas. Certain areas may be more relevant for certain users. For example, the section on physical examination may be particularly useful for clinical geneticist physicians. Many questions might be assigned to multiple areas, however – that is, some questions span multiple themes.

Second, the questions cover multiple different areas of genetics. Depending on a person's level of training and experience, some questions may seem laughably easy, while others may be much trickier.

Third, I have tried to keep the questions short and straightforward so that learners would not get tripped up by semantics. This may mean that some questions may not perfectly mirror the style used in examinations, though examination style can differ and change with time and examination type. Although some examinations now shy away from "all of the above" and similar question formats (despite Maino's excellent song), I have retained a few of these types of questions here, as I feel that they can be useful when studying.

Fourth, related to the above point, I have kept the answers clear and succinct. Rather than exploring at length the reasons why all the choices given in the multiple choice questions are correct or incorrect, I provide a short explanation focusing on the correct answer. Based on my own experience, and from talking to colleagues, I have found that overly long discussions can be somewhat distracting, and bogs learners down when the idea is to expose them to information about many different concepts and conditions.

Finally, I have endeavored to make the information as "future-proof" as possible so that this book will not quickly become obsolete. Along these lines, the references include many traditional scientific and medical articles and textbooks, as well as online articles and other web-based resources. I anticipate that some of these latter references may change with time, and I encourage readers who want to delve deeper into a particular topic to check the latest literature.

For those looking for new questions after completing this book, you can follow me on Twitter (@BenjaminSolomo2). Best of luck, and thanks for your interest!

Basics and Terminology

1

1.1. Both a child and the child's mother are affected by the same genetic condition, but the child is more severely affected. Which of the following terms best describes this scenario?

A. Allelic heterogeneity
B. Incomplete penetrance
C. Pleiotropy
D. Variable expressivity

1.2. About how many protein-coding genes are there in the human genome?

A. 9000
B. 19 000
C. 90 000
D. 900 000

1.3. Which of the following refers to the most common isochromosome in humans?

A. i(1q)
B. i(18p)
C. i(Xq)
D. i(Yp)

1.4. A patient has undergone extensive genetic testing without finding an explanation for their health condition. They enroll in a research study involving a new type of genomic analysis. As part of enrollment, informed consent is obtained. What basic ethical principle includes informed consent?

A. Beneficence
B. Justice
C. Respect for persons
D. Subject selection

1.5. What best describes the following genetic change: c.1138G>A?

A. Transcription
B. Transition
C. Translation
D. Transversion

1.6. Holt-Oram syndrome, due to pathogenic variants in the gene *TBX5*, can include both limb and heart anomalies. What term best explains the fact that this condition affects multiple organ systems?

A. Contiguous gene syndrome
B. Epigenetics
C. Incomplete penetrance
D. Pleiotropy

1.7. Approximately what percentage of the human genome does the exome represent?

A. 0.01%
B. 1%
C. 10%
D. 100%

1.8. Approximately how many base pairs are in the haploid human genome?

A. 1 million
B. 1 billion
C. 3 billion
D. 3 trillion

1.9. What best describes the following in humans: LINE-1, SVA, and Alu?

A. Active mobile elements
B. Gene therapy
C. HOX genes
D. Immunotherapeutics

Medical Genetics and Genomics: Questions for Board Review, First Edition. Benjamin D. Solomon.
© 2023 John Wiley & Sons Ltd. Published 2023 by John Wiley & Sons Ltd.

1.10. Which germ layer gives rise to the central nervous system?
A. Ectoderm
B. Endoderm
C. Mesoderm
D. Homeoderm

1.11. What is the term for the type of DNA modifications that do not alter the DNA sequence, but which can affect the activity of a gene?
A. Epigenetic
B. Homeostatic
C. Lentiviral
D. Silent

1.12. Approximately how many kb of DNA are included in mitochondrial DNA (mtDNA)?
A. 0.01 kb
B. 1.4 kb
C. 16.5 kb
D. 250 kb

1.13. The centromeres of human chromosomes 13, 14, 15, 21, and 22 are located near one end of the chromosomes. What type of chromosomes are these?
A. Acrocentric
B. Metacentric
C. Submetacentric
D. Telocentric

1.14. Which of the following is NOT a DNA nucleotide base?
A. Adenine
B. Cytosine
C. Thymine
D. Uracil

1.15. During meiosis, when does recombination (crossing-over) occur?
A. Meiosis I
B. Meiosis II
C. Mitosis
D. Cytokinesis

1.16. What is the term for the caudal displacement and herniation of the cerebellar structures into the cervical spinal canal?
A. Anencephaly
B. Ectopia cordis
C. Chiari malformation
D. Tethered cord

1.17. To try to determine the cause of a patient's condition, researchers decide to analyze the patient's transcriptome. In the planned transcriptome sequencing, what will be interrogated?
A. DNA
B. Metabolites
C. Proteins
D. RNA

1.18. Which term refers to the nonrandom co-occurrence of clinical features, but without the implication of a single underlying/unifying cause?
A. Association
B. Dysplasia
C. Sequence
D. Syndrome

1.19. Which of the following is NOT a stop codon?
A. UAA
B. UAG
C. UGA
D. UGG

1.20. What is the term for the byproduct of meiosis in oocytes?
A. Barr body
B. Chiasmata
C. Polar body
D. Telomere

1.21. What is the smallest human chromosome?
A. 1
B. 21
C. 22
D. X

1.22. A patient has signs of a specific genetic condition; genetic sequencing reveals a variant for which there is strong evidence of disease causation. The variant is present in the patient and other affected family members (but not unaffected family members). This variant has been identified in other, unrelated individuals with the same condition (but not unaffected individuals). There is functional and computational support for disease causation. Which term would be the best for this variant?

   A. A mutation   **C.** A pathogenic variant
   B. A polymorphism   **D.** Wild type

1.23. Which of the following is the best term for insufficient (but not absent) cellular proliferation?

   A. Aplasia   **C.** Dysplasia
   B. Atrophy   **D.** Hypoplasia

1.24. A person has had genetic testing; the following genetic change was identified and mentioned in a clinical note: m.8944A>G. What kind of variant is this?

   A. Marker chromosome   **C.** Mitochondrial
   B. Maternal   **D.** Monoallelic

1.25. Which term describes failure of the lower limbs to form separately?

   A. Hemihypertrophy   **C.** Polydactyly
   B. Macrosomia   **D.** Sirenomelia

1.26. Which of the following refers to the presence of a mixture of different cells, with different genetic information, in a person?

   A. Aneuploidy   **C.** Heterozygosity
   B. Deletion   **D.** Mosaicism

1.27. There are many known different genetic causes (involving different genes) of dilated cardiomyopathy. What is the best term for this phenomenon?

   A. Allelic heterogeneity   **C.** Incomplete penetrance
   B. Genetic heterogeneity   **D.** Pleiotropism

1.28. About what percent of DNA is considered to be noncoding DNA?

   A. 1%   **C.** 49%
   B. 25%   **D.** 99%

1.29. Which of the following refers to a collection of neurons that have not migrated to their normal position?

   A. Heterotopia   **C.** Lissencephaly
   B. Hydranencephaly   **D.** Pachygyria

1.30. Different pathogenic variants in the gene *LMNA* can result in a number of different/distinct genetic conditions. These conditions might be referred to as which of the following (i.e. how would these conditions relate to each other)?

   A. Allelic conditions   **C.** Polygenic conditions
   B. Oligogenic conditions   **D.** Recessive conditions

1.31. Which of the following is the last phase of mitosis?

   A. Anaphase   **C.** Prophase
   B. Metaphase   **D.** Telophase

1.32. What is the term for the process by which the information stored in the DNA is transferred to RNA?
A. Cytokinesis
B. Replication
C. Transcription
D. Translation

1.33. Chromothripsis might be described as a form of which of the following?
A. Cardiac anomaly
B. Gene therapy
C. Genomic instability
D. Meiosis

1.34. Which of the following terms refers to portions of DNA, or the corresponding sections of an RNA transcript, that are translated into protein?
A. Exon
B. Gene
C. Intron
D. Polypeptide

1.35. Which of the following hypothetical protein changes would indicate a nonsense variant (mutation)?
A. p.Trp321Cys
B. p.Trp321Ter or p.Trp321*
C. c.321A>C
D. p.Trp321=

1.36. What is the term for cells that have a mixture of mitochondria containing "mutated" and wild-type DNA?
A. Compound heterozygous
B. Heteroplasmic
C. Homoplasmic
D. Variably expressed

1.37. A patient is found to have fluid-filled cysts in the brain. Which is the correct term for this finding?
A. Cephalohematoma
B. Craniosynostosis
C. Porencephaly
D. Schizencephaly

1.38. A genetic variant is written as: c.7950T>C (p.Asn2650=)
What's the best description of this variant at the protein level?
A. Deletion
B. Missense
C. Nonsense
D. Silent

1.39. What is the term for the "constriction" in a chromosome, which separates the long and short arms of the chromosome?
A. Centromere
B. Cytokinesis
C. Fragile site
D. Telomere

1.40. Which of the following provides structural support for chromosomes?
A. Golgi body
B. Histone
C. Lysosome
D. Peroxisome

1.41. Which of the following best describes the structure of DNA?
A. Beta-pleated sheet
B. Left-handed double helix
C. Right-handed double helix
D. Triple helix

1.42. Which of the following is an autosome?
A. Centromere
B. Chromosome 1
C. X chromosome
D. Y chromosome

1.43. Which of the following refers to the study or analysis of genetic material from a mixed community of organisms, such as different microbes?

    A. Epigenetics   **C.** Proteomics

    B. Metagenomics   **D.** Transcriptomics

1.44. Which organelle or part of the cell serves as the site of protein synthesis in the cell?

    A. Lysosome   **C.** Peroxisome

    B. Nucleus   **D.** Ribosome

1.45. CRISPR-Cas9 is a gene-editing technique that is adapted from a naturally occurring-system in what type of organism?

    A. Bacteria   **C.** Fungi

    B. Drosophila   **D.** Virus

1.46. Which of the following is NOT transcribed?

    A. 3′UTR   **C.** Intron

    B. Exon   **D.** Promoter

1.47. Which of the following is a term for X-inactivation?

    A. Compound heterozygosity   **C.** Mosaicism

    B. Lyonization   **D.** RNA interference

1.48. A genetic variant is indicated as follows: NM_006735.4(HOXA2):c.394T>A (p.Ser132Thr) Which part of this phrasing refers to the specific genetic change in the reference sequence of the coding DNA?

    A. NM_006735.4   **C.** c.394T>A

    B. HOXA2   **D.** p.Ser132Thr

1.49. Which of the following terms describes decreased skull mineralization?

    A. Craniosynostosis   **C.** Cutis aplasia

    B. Craniotabes   **D.** Osteopetrosis

1.50. Two different, genetically distinguishable populations interbreed and have off-spring, who have a mix of genetic information from the two populations. Which best describes "mixing" of genetic information in this way?

    A. Admixture   **C.** Homology

    B. Consanguinity   **D.** Recombination

1.51. Which of the following genes is considered to be a tumor suppressor gene?

    A. *EGFR*   **C.** *RET*

    B. *ERBB*   **D.** *TP53*

1.52. Which of the following refers to a chromosome with two centromeres, and which contains mirror-image segments of genetic material?

    A. Acrocentric   **C.** Euchromatic

    B. Aneuploid   **D.** Isodicentric

1.53. Which term refers to the process of programmed cell death?

    A. Apoptosis   **C.** Hypoplasia

    B. Cytokinesis   **D.** Lysis

1.54. Which type of RNA recognizes and carries specific amino acids to the ribosomes for assembly into protein chains?

A. mRNA

B. rRNA

C. snRNA

D. tRNA

1.55. Which of the following would represent a frameshift variant?

A. c.169_170insA

B. c.79_80delinsTT

C. g.123A>G

D. p.Trp24Cys

1.56. Approximately what percentage of the human genome consists of repetitive elements?

A. 10%

B. 25%

C. 50%

D. 99%

1.57. Which of the following is a membrane-bound organelle that contains digestive enzymes and is involved in a number of cellular processes, including apoptosis, metabolism of large molecules, and destruction of pathogens?

A. Golgi body

B. Lysosome

C. Mitochondrion

D. Ribosome

1.58. The Genetic Information Nondiscrimination Act (GINA) of 2008 aims to protect Americans from discrimination based on their genetic information related to which of the choices below?

A. Disability insurance and life insurance

B. Employment

C. Health insurance and employment

D. Long-term care insurance

1.59. Which of the following refers to a sequence of DNA that closely resembles a gene, but which has become (apparently) inactive through evolution, and which can result in challenges in genetic testing?

A. Euchromatin

B. Haplotype

C. Pseudogene

D. Recombinant DNA

1.60. In humans, autosomal aneuploidies are overall most commonly due to what type of meiotic error?

A. Maternal meiosis I

B. Maternal meiosis II

C. Paternal meiosis I

D. Paternal meiosis II

Answers

Basics and terminology

1.1. D	**1.8.** C	**1.15.** A	**1.22.** C
1.2. B	**1.9.** A	**1.16.** C	**1.23.** D
1.3. C	**1.10.** A	**1.17.** D	**1.24.** C
1.4. C	**1.11.** A	**1.18.** A	**1.25.** D
1.5. B	**1.12.** C	**1.19.** D	**1.26.** D
1.6. D	**1.13.** A	**1.20.** C	**1.27.** B
1.7. B	**1.14.** D	**1.21.** B	**1.28.** D

1.29.	A	1.37.	C	1.45.	A	1.53.	A
1.30.	A	1.38.	D	1.46.	D	1.54.	D
1.31.	D	1.39.	A	1.47.	B	1.55.	A
1.32.	C	1.40.	B	1.48.	C	1.56.	C
1.33.	C	1.41.	C	1.49.	B	1.57.	B
1.34.	A	1.42.	B	1.50.	A	1.58.	C
1.35.	B	1.43.	B	1.51.	D	1.59.	C
1.36.	B	1.44.	D	1.52.	D	1.60.	A

Commentary

1.1. Variable expressivity

Variable expressivity refers to the range of clinical manifestations that can occur in different people with the same genetic condition. In the question, both the child and the mother are affected by the condition but are differently affected. Penetrance, on the other hand, is the proportion of people that have a certain genetic change who have clinical manifestations of a genetic disorder. Incomplete penetrance means that not all people with the given genetic change have clinical manifestations – that is, some are unaffected.

Reference(s): Nussbaum et al. [1].

1.2. 19 000

It is currently estimated that there are about 19 000 protein-coding genes in the human genome. Over the past several decades, this estimate has decreased. Prior to the first sequencing of the human genome, estimates fell in the 40 000–100 000 range; after the human genome was first sequenced, that number was revised to about 26 000–30 000. More recent proteomic and evolutionary studies have further decreased the estimate to the 19 000–20 000 range. Additional genes have been identified through newer endeavors that aimed to sequence and analyze regions that were previously difficult to interrogate.

Reference(s): Lander et al., [2]; Clamp et al. [3]; Ezkurdia et al. [4].

1.3. i(Xq)

The term "isochromosome" refers to a chromosome that results from duplication of part of a chromosome and deletion of the non-duplicated part. This yields a chromosome that is a mirror image copy of the duplicated chromosomal region. There are multiple types of isochromosomes; the type depends on where on the chromosome the chromosomal break occurs. The most common isochromosome affects the long arm of the X chromosome and is written using standard nomenclature as: i(Xq).

Reference(s): Gonzaga-Jauregui and Lupski [5].

1.4. Respect for persons

The Belmont Report, which derived from formal commissioned work in the 1970s, describes the basic ethical principles that should underlie biomedical and behavioral research involving human subjects. The Belmont Report also developed guidelines based on these principles. The three basic ethical principles described are respect for persons; beneficence; justice. Per the report, "respect for persons incorporates at least two ethical convictions: first, that individuals should be treated as autonomous agents, and second, that persons with diminished autonomy are entitled to protection." Though there are many nuances, including as relates to genomic research, informed consent is considered to be part of respect for persons.

Reference(s): Mathews and Jamal [6]; The Belmont Report [7].

1.5. Transition

A transition describes a genetic variant where a purine (adenine or guanine) is changed to another purine or a pyrimidine (cytosine or thymine) is changed to another pyrimidine. A transversion describes a change from a purine to a pyrimidine or vice versa.

Reference(s): Nussbaum et al. [1].

1.6. Pleiotropy

The term pleiotropy means that a change in a certain gene results in multiple, apparently unrelated, manifestations in an affected person. In the example given, heterozygous pathogenic variants in the gene *TBX5* cause Holt-Oram syndrome, which can include upper limb anomalies, as well as structural cardiac and cardiac conduction anomalies.

Reference(s): Paaby and Rockman [8]; McDermott et al. [9].

1.7. 1%

The exome refers to the protein-coding portions, or exons, of the genes. Current estimates suggest that there are about 19 000 genes in the human genome. The exome makes up about 1–2% of the human genome. Exome sequencing has emerged as a powerful tool in the diagnosis of many genetic conditions.

Reference(s): Ng et al. [10]; Ezkurdia et al. [4]; Biesecker and Green [11].

1.8. Three billion

The haploid human genome contains approximately 3 billion base pairs. That is, people inherit about 3 billion base pairs of DNA from each parent, so the diploid human genome, arranged on 23 pairs of chromosomes, totals approximately 6 billion base pairs.

Reference(s): Lander et al. [2]; National Human Genome Research Institute: The Human Genome Project Completion [12].

1.9. Active mobile elements

LINE-1 (L1), SVAs, and Alus represent three types of active mobile elements in humans. Mobile element insertions (MEIs) can cause disease through a number of mechanisms, including insertional mutagenesis and aberrant splicing, as well as due to deletions at the insertion site, all of which can disrupt normal gene function. In addition to implications related to evolution and related areas, MEIs may represent an underappreciated but clinically important type of pathogenic variant in genetic testing.

Reference(s): Cordaux and Batzer [13]; Kazazian and Moran [14]; Torene et al. [15].

1.10. Ectoderm

Gastrulation occurs during the third week of gestation in humans and includes establishment of the three germ layers: ectoderm, endoderm, and mesoderm. Different structures and organ systems arise from each of these germ layers during the process of development. Structures eventually formed from the ectoderm include the adrenal medulla, cornea, central nervous system, hair and nails, peripheral nervous system, sensory epithelia, pituitary, subcutaneous glands, and tooth enamel. Structures eventually formed from the endoderm include the epithelial lining of the gastrointestinal and respiratory tracts and bladder/urethra, as well as portions of the liver, pancreas, parathyroid, thyroid, and tonsils. Structures eventually formed from the mesoderm include the adrenal cortex, blood and lymphatic vessels, bone, cartilage, connective tissue, gonads, heart, serous membranes lining the body cavities, skeletal muscle, and spleen.

Reference(s): Moore and Persaud [16].

1.11. Epigenetic

Epigenetic changes refer to DNA modifications that do not change the actual DNA sequence, but which can still affect a gene's activity and may therefore affect human health. Epigenetic mechanisms have long been recognized as contributors to certain disorders; recent evidence shows that these epigenetic mechanisms may contribute more substantially to a wider group of congenital (as well as other) conditions.

Reference(s): Egger et al. [17]; Barbosa et al. [18].

1.12. 16.5 kb

The mitochondrial DNA (mtDNA) includes 16.5 kb (16 500 base pairs) of DNA. This DNA includes 37 genes, 13 of which encode enzymes involved in oxidative phosphorylation. Separate from the mtDNA, the nuclear genome encodes over 1000 mitochondrial proteins. Pathogenic variants affecting the mtDNA can result in a variety of clinical conditions.

Reference(s): Schon et al. [19]; Chinnery [20].

1.13. Acrocentric

Chromosomes may be described by the location of the centromeres. The centromeres of acrocentric chromosomes are located near one end of the chromosome. In humans, chromosomes 13, 14, 15, 21, and 22 are acrocentric chromosomes.

Reference(s): Nussbaum et al. [1].

1.14. Uracil

DNA is made up of four different units, or nucleotide bases. The DNA bases are adenine (A), cytosine (C), guanine (G), and thymine (T). RNA also has four bases: adenine, cytosine, guanine, and uracil (U).

Reference(s): Nussbaum et al. [1]; National Human Genome Research Institute: A Brief Guide to Genomics [21].

1.15. Meiosis I

During meiosis, haploid gametes (egg and sperm) are formed from diploid cells. Through meiosis, four gametes are formed from each parent cell, and each gamete has half the number of chromosomes compared to the parent cell. Meiosis includes a round of DNA synthesis and two rounds of chromosome segregation and cell division (Meiosis I and Meiosis II). Within each round of meiosis, there are multiple steps. Recombination occurs during meiosis I.

Reference(s): Moore [16]; Nussbaum et al. [1].

1.16. Chiari malformation

A Chiari malformation (or Arnold-Chiari malformation) refers to caudal displacement and herniation of the cerebellar structures into the cervical spinal canal. Multiple types and categories have been described. Overall, Chiari malformations can occur in an apparently isolated fashion or as part of a syndromic presentation.

Reference(s): Stevenson et al. [22].

1.17. RNA

There are multiple types of testing that may reveal the cause of a patient's genetic disorder. These may include biochemical, cytogenomic, molecular, and other tests. In some patients, transcriptome sequencing has been able to identify answers. The transcriptome refers to all of the expressed RNA molecules. Transcriptome sequencing can provide information about gene activity in a cell or tissue. Often, results are correlated with DNA-based or other assays to try to arrive at a definitive diagnosis.

Reference(s): Cummings et al. [23]; Frésard et al. [24].

1.18. Association

An association refers to nonrandom co-occurrence of multiple clinical features (that is these features occur together more often than would be expected by chance alone), but without the implication of a single underlying/unifying cause. An example of a condition that is currently considered to be an association is VACTERL association.

Reference(s): Stevenson et al. [22].

1.19. UGG

A codon refers to a set of three adjacent mRNA bases that encode an amino acid or termination of translation. The three stop (or nonsense) codons are: UAA, UAG, UGA. That is, these three codons designate the stoppage (termination) of translation.

Reference(s): Nussbaum et al. [1].

1.20. Polar body

Polar bodies are haploid cells that are formed as a byproduct of oocyte meiotic division. Polar bodies form during both rounds of meiosis. Ordinarily, polar bodies are not fertilized and undergo apoptosis.

Reference(s): Schmerler and Wessel [25].

1.21. 21

The smallest human chromosome is chromosome 21. Chromosome 21 includes about 48 million base pairs, which is about 2% of the genome. By comparison, chromosome 1, the largest human chromosome, includes about 249 million base pairs, or about 8% of the genome. Although the chromosomes are generally ordered in terms of size, chromosome 21 is numbered prior to chromosome 22 because the former appeared larger using conventional cytogenetic techniques (prior to the sequencing of the chromosomes).

Reference(s): Lander et al. [2]; Genetics Home Reference [26].

1.22. Pathogenic variant

There are different ways to describe genetic changes. One system describes variants in terms of clinical significance (e.g. benign variant, likely benign variant, variant of uncertain significance, likely pathogenic variant, pathogenic variant). This system relies on multiple lines of evidence, including prevalence in affected and unaffected populations, familial segregation data, and functional/biologic data. Of the choices in the question, "pathogenic variant" would be the most accurate description.

Reference(s): Richard et al. [27]; Jarvik and Evans [28].

1.23. Hypoplasia

Hypoplasia refers to insufficient cellular proliferation. This reduction in cell proliferation leads to deficient tissue mass and undergrowth of the affected organ or morphologic feature.

Reference(s): Stevenson et al. [22].

1.24. Mitochondrial

The variant mentioned in the question includes the prefix "m." This means that this is a mitochondrial variant (a variant that occurs in the mitochondrial reference sequence). Many different clinically relevant medical conditions can result from mitochondrial variants.

Reference(s): den Dunnen [29].

1.25. Sirenomelia

Sirenomelia is a lower limb malformation that refers to failure of the lower limbs to form separately. As with other congenital anomalies, there is a range of severity. Sirenomelia is almost always accompanied by vascular and other major malformations. The overall causes are not well understood, but there is evidence of association with factors such as maternal diabetes mellitus, young maternal age, and twin gestations.

Reference(s): Orioli et al. [30]; Boer et al. [31]; Stevenson et al. [22].

1.26. Mosaicism

Mosaicism refers to the presence of multiple different cells with different genetic information (genotypes) occurring in a person. There are several different types of mosaicism. Being able to determine whether genetic variants are mosaic can be clinically important.

Reference(s): Biesecker and Spinner [32]; Stosser et al. [33].

1.27. Genetic heterogeneity

Dilated cardiomyopathy can be caused by pathogenic variants in many different genes. This phenomenon, in which there can be many different genetic causes for a condition, is known as genetic heterogeneity. Many conditions demonstrate genetic heterogeneity. In contrast, allelic heterogeneity refers to different pathogenic variants at the same genetic locus (typically meaning the same gene) causing the same condition.

Reference(s): McClellan and King [34]; Jordan and Hershberger [35].

1.28. 99%

About 99% of a person's DNA is noncoding DNA – it does not include protein-coding genes. Noncoding DNA contains regulatory elements, instructions for certain RNA molecules, and structural elements. Much remains to be understood about the function of noncoding DNA.

Reference(s): ENCODE project consortium [36]; Genetics Home Reference [26].

1.29. Heterotopia

A heterotopia refers to a collection of neurons that have not migrated to their normal position. There are multiple types of heterotopias. Heterotopias can be associated with seizures and may occur in the context of a known genetic disorder or syndrome, or in an apparently isolated context.

Reference(s): Watrin et al. [37]; Romero et al. [38]; Stevenson et al. [22].

1.30. Allelic conditions

Distinct conditions may be referred to as "allelic conditions" when they are caused by different pathogenic variants in the same gene. For example, many distinct conditions may be caused by pathogenic variants in the gene *LMNA*. These include Charcot-Marie-Tooth disease, dilated cardiomyopathy, Emery-Dreifuss muscular dystrophy, Hutchinson-Gilford Progeria, and Mandibuloacral dysplasia. In general, while allelic conditions involve the same gene, the underlying biological mechanism may be different (and may involve variants in different functional domains or with different inheritance patterns), which results in distinct phenotypes. There can also be controversy over whether conditions are truly allelic or whether they represent a disease spectrum or continuum.

Reference(s): Ho and Hegele [39]; Nussbaum et al. [1].

1.31. Telophase

Mitosis is the process through which one cell divides to become two genetically identical "daughter cells." Mitosis has four main phases, which occur in the following order: prophase, metaphase, anaphase, telophase. Cytokinesis, in which the cell contents are divided, starts in anaphase or telophase.

Reference(s): Nussbaum et al. [1].

1.32. Transcription

The information stored in a gene's DNA is transferred to RNA during the process of transcription. The process of translation involves the stage at which RNA is translated to protein.

Reference(s): Nussbaum et al. [1].

1.33. Genomic instability

Chromothripsis, a form of genomic instability, is a mutational phenomenon where tens to hundreds of locally clustered genomic arrangements typically occur all at once. Chromothripsis can be relevant to cancer, as well as to congenital disorders.

Reference(s): Stephens et al. [40]; Zhang et al. [41]; Cortes-Ciriano et al. [42].

1.34. Exon

An exon refers to portions of DNA, or the corresponding sections of an RNA transcript, that are translated into protein.

Reference(s): Scitable [43].

1.35. p.Trp321Ter or p.Trp321*

"p.Trp321Ter" or "p.Trp321*" indicates that the amino acid "Trp" (an abbreviation for the amino acid tryptophan, which is also sometimes abbreviated with the single letter "W"), located at position 321 has been changed to a stop codon, denoted by "Ter" or "*".

Reference(s): den Dunnen [29].

1.36. Heteroplasmic

Heteroplasmy is the term for cells with a mixture of mitochondria; some mutated, and some not. This concept is important clinically, including to help counsel patients who may be suspected or known to have a mitochondrial condition. As the level of heteroplasmy in a given tissue increases, a threshold may be reached at which a phenotypic or clinical effect may be observed. The level of heteroplasmy may differ from one tissue to the next.

Reference(s): Freyer et al. [44]; Stewart and Chinnery [45].

1.37. Porencephaly

Porencephaly refers to the presence of fluid-filled cysts in the brain. The severity of the condition can be highly variable. There are genetic conditions that can cause porencephaly, which can occur in syndromic and non-syndromic contexts.

Reference(s): Yoneda et al. [46]; Del Guidice et al. [47].

1.38. Silent

A silent variant is a change in the DNA sequence that does not change the amino acid sequence of the encoded protein.

Reference(s): den Dunnen [29].

1.39. Centromere

The centromere refers to a "constriction" in the chromosome, and separates the chromosome into the short and long arms. Replication occurs in cell division, resulting in sister chromatids. These sister chromatids are joined at the centromere.

Reference(s): National Human Genome Research Institute Talking Glossary of Genetics Terms [48].

1.40. Histone

DNA is a very long molecule and is packaged in a specific way in the cell nucleus. As part of the packaging process, DNA wraps around proteins called histones. Histones provide structural support for the chromosome, thus allowing DNA to be packed compactly. Histones can also be involved in regulation of gene expression.

Reference(s): National Human Genome Research Institute Talking Glossary of Genetics Terms [49].

1.41. Right-handed double helix

DNA is a double-stranded molecule that forms a helical spiral. "Normal" DNA forms a right-handed double helix, meaning the twisting appears to be clockwise when viewed from the end. There are also rare forms of DNA that are left-handed.

Reference(s): Watson and Crick [50]; Mitsui et al. [51]; Wang [52].

1.42. Chromosome 1

Humans have 23 pairs of chromosomes, of which there are 22 pairs of autosomes and one pair of sex chromosomes. The autosomes consist of the "numbered chromosomes" (all of the chromosomes except the X and Y chromosomes).

Reference(s): National Human Genome Research Institute Talking Glossary of Genetic Terms [53].

1.43. Metagenomics

Metagenomics refers to the study of genetic material derived from a mixed community of organisms. In practice, this often refers to sequencing and analyzing the DNA or RNA of multiple microbial species (and host organisms) taken from a certain source or sources.

Reference(s): Chiu and Miller [54].

1.44. Ribosome

Ribosomes, which are made of RNA and protein, are the sites for protein synthesis in the cell. That is, ribosomes translate the sequence of messenger RNA (mRNA) to polypeptide chains.

Reference(s): Steitz [55]; National Human Genome Research Institute Talking Glossary of Genetic Terms [56].

1.45. Bacteria

A number of different gene editing techniques are being used to address a variety of research questions. CRISPR-Cas9, one such gene editing technique, has been adapted from a naturally occurring system that bacteria use to combat viruses.

Reference(s): Doudna and Charpentier [57]; Adli [58].

1.46. Promoter

The promoter (or promoter region) is a type of DNA regulatory element. Typically, the promoter is located just upstream or next to the place where a gene will be transcribed.

Reference(s): Andersson and Sandelin [59]; Nussbaum et al. [1]; National Human Genome Research Institute Talking Glossary of Genetic Terms [60].

1.47. Lyonization

X-inactivation, sometimes called Lyonization (after the geneticist Mary Lyon), refers to the process by which a copy of genes on the X-chromosome are "turned off" in female mammals. This occurs due to transcriptional silencing, which is controlled by the X-inactivation center.

Reference(s): Avner and Heard [61]; Galupa and Heard [62]; National Human Genome Research Institute Talking Glossary of Genetic Terms [59].

1.48. c.394T>A

To help provide clarity and uniformity, there is recommended specific nomenclature regarding how to describe genetic variants. In this example, NM_006735.4 refers to the coding DNA reference sequence, HOXA2 refers to the name of the gene, c.394T>A refers to the specific genetic change in the coding DNA reference sequence, and p.Ser132Thr refers to the change in the protein reference sequence.

Reference(s): den Dunnen [29].

1.49. Craniotabes

Craniotabes refer to decreased skull mineralization, which results in abnormal softness of the skull. Craniotabes can occur in a number of different genetic conditions and syndromes that involve abnormal mineralization, but can also be due to nongenetic causes.

Reference(s): Eldrissy [63]; Stevenson et al. [22].

1.50. Admixture

In genetics, admixture (or genetic admixture) occurs when individuals from genetically distinguishable groups reproduce. The offspring of these groups will have genetic information from each of the populations. Information regarding genetic admixture can be helpful to address many different research and clinically oriented questions.

Reference(s): Meyer et al. [64]; Hellenthal et al. [65].

1.51. *TP53*

Tumor suppressor genes encode proteins involved in processes such as slowing cell division, repairing DNA, or triggering cell death. Variants in tumor suppressor genes can lead to uncontrolled cell growth, which can contribute to cancer. *TP53* is an example of a tumor suppressor gene.

Reference(s): Rivlin et al. [66]; Schneider et al. [67].

1.52. Isodicentric

There are many different types of chromosomal rearrangements and anomalies. An isodicentric chromosome has two centromeres (instead of the normal single centromere) and contains mirror-image segments of DNA. Isodicentric chromosomes can be involved with or result in genetic disorders, including related to congenital, as well as oncologic conditions.

Reference(s): Nakagome et al. [68]; Tuck-Muller et al. [69]; Lusk et al. [70].

1.53. Apoptosis

Apoptosis refers to the process of programmed cell death. Apoptosis is important in key developmental and other health and disease-related processes, such as cancer. Certain genes/proteins are particularly important in the regulation of apoptosis.

Reference(s): Elmore [71]; Singh et al. [72]; National Human Genome Research Institute Talking Glossary of Genetic Terms [73].

1.54. tRNA

There are several kinds of ribonucleic acid (RNA), each of which performs different functions. Among these types, transfer RNA (trNA) recognizes specific amino acids and brings them to the ribosomes to be assembled into protein chains. Other types of RNA include messenger RNA (mRNA) and ribosomal RNA (rRNA).

Reference(s): National Human Genome Research Institute Talking Glossary of Genetic Terms [74].

1.55. c.169_170insA

A frameshift variant involves the insertion or deletion of a number of base pairs that is not a multiple of three. This change alters the DNA sequence's triplet reading frame, and usually results in a truncated protein product due to a premature stop codon.

Reference(s): den Dunnen [29].

1.56. 50%

Repetitive elements are found frequently in the genomes of both prokaryotes and eukaryotes. It is estimated that about half of the human genome consists of repetitive elements. However, estimates vary considerably. Though challenging to accurately sequence and analyze, there is growing evidence that variants in these repetitive elements can contribute to a number of different human diseases, including in complex ways.

Reference(s): Haubold and Wiehle [75]; Tannan [76]; Mitra et al. [77].

1.57. Lysosome

Lysosomes are membrane-bound organelles that contain digestive enzymes. Lysosomes are involved in many cellular processes, including the metabolism of large molecules, destruction of pathogens, and apoptosis. A number of genetic conditions are considered lysosomal disorders, including Batten disease, cystinosis, Fabry disease, Gaucher disease, mucolipidoses, mucopolysaccharide storage diseases, and Pompe disease, to name just a few of the more than 50 different conditions.

Reference(s): Staretz-Chacham et al. [78]; Lachmann [79]; National Human Genome Research Institute Talking Glossary of Genetic Terms [80].

1.58. Health insurance and employment

A number of different laws help guide and regulate issues related to genetics and genomics, including how this information can be used in different situations. In the United States, the Genetic Information Nondiscrimination Act (GINA), enacted in 2008, helps provide protection from discrimination based on a person's genetic information as relates to health insurance and employment.

Reference(s): McGuire and Majumder [81]; Lenartz et al. [82]; National Human Genome Research Institute: Policy Issues in Genomics [83].

1.59. Pseudogene

A pseudogene is a sequence of DNA that closely resembles a gene, but which has become (apparently) inactive through evolution. The presence of pseudogenes can cause challenges in genetic testing processes; for example, it can be difficult to determine if a detected variant occurs in a gene or a similar pseudogene.

Reference(s): Song et al. [84]; National Human Genome Research Institute Talking Glossary of Genetic Terms [85].

1.60. Maternal meiosis I

Human aneuploidies are relatively common. Overall, the meiotic event giving rise to autosomal aneuploidies most commonly occurs during maternal meiosis I. However, the proportion of when and where the event occurs varies according to the particular aneuploidy. That is, depending on the particular aneuploidy, the event may occur during maternal meiosis II or during paternal meiosis I or II or postzygotic mitosis.

Reference(s): Hassold and Hunt [86].

References

1. Nussbaum, R.L., McInnes, R.R., and Willard, H.F. (2016). *Thompson & Thompson Genetics in Medicine*. Philadelphia, PA: Elsevier.
2. Lander, E.S., Linton, L.M., Birren, B. et al. (2001). Initial sequencing and analysis of the human genome. *Nature* 409: 860–921.

3. Clamp, M., Fry, B., Kamal, M. et al. (2007). Distinguishing protein-coding and noncoding genes in the human genome. *Proc. Natl Acad. Sci. USA* 104: 19428–19433.

4. Ezkurdia, I., Juan, D., Rodriguez, J.M. et al. (2014). Multiple evidence strands suggest that there may be as few as 19,000 human protein-coding genes. *Hum. Mol. Genet.* 23: 5866–5878.

5. Gonzaga-Jauregui, C. and Lupski, J.R. (2021). *Genomics of Rare Diseases: Understanding Disease Genetics Using Genomic Approaches*. San Diego, CA: Academic Press.

6. Mathews, D.J. and Jamal, L. (2014). Revisiting respect for persons in genomic research. *Genes* 5: 1–12.

7. The Belmont Report. https://www.hhs.gov/ohrp/regulations-and-policy/belmont-report/index.html (accessed July 26, 2021).

8. Paaby, A.B. and Rockman, M.V. (2013). The many faces of pleiotropy. *Trends Genet.* 29: 66–73.

9. McDermott, D.A., Fong, J.C., and Basson, C.T. (1993). Holt-Oram syndrome. In: *Gene Reviews*® (ed. M.P. Adam, H.H. Ardinger, R.A. Pagon, et al.). Seattle, WA: University of Washington.

10. Ng, S.B., Buckingham, K.J., Lee, C. et al. (2010). Exome sequencing identifies the cause of a mendelian disorder. *Nat. Genet.* 42: 30–35.

11. Biesecker, L.G. and Green, R.C. (2014). Diagnostic clinical genome and exome sequencing. *N. Engl. J. Med.* 370: 2418–2425.

12. Human Genome Project FAQ. https://www.genome.gov/11006943/human-genome-project-completion-frequently-asked-questions/ (accessed 26 July 2021).

13. Cordaux, R. and Batzer, M.A. (2009). The impact of retrotransposons on human genome evolution. *Nat. Rev. Genet.* 10: 691–703.

14. Kazazian, H.H. Jr. and Moran, J.V. (2017). Mobile DNA in health and disease. *N. Engl. J. Med.* 377: 361–370.

15. Torene, R.I., Galens, K., Liu, S. et al. (2020). Mobile element insertion detection in 89,874 clinical exomes. *Genet. Med.* 22: 974–978.

16. Moore, K.L. (2020). *The Developing Human: Clinically Oriented Embryology*. Edinburgh; New York: Elsevier.

17. Egger, G., Liang, G., Aparicio, A., and Jones, P.A. (2004). Epigenetics in human disease and prospects for epigenetic therapy. *Nature* 429: 457–463.

18. Barbosa, M., Joshi, R.S., Garg, P. et al. (2018). Identification of rare de novo epigenetic variations in congenital disorders. *Nat. Commun.* 9: 2064.

19. Schon, E.A., DiMauro, S., and Hirano, M. (2012). Human mitochondrial DNA: roles of inherited and somatic mutations. *Nat. Rev. Genet.* 13: 878–890.

20. Chinnery, P.F. (1993). Primary mitochondrial disorders overview. In: *GeneReviews*® (ed. M.P. Adam, H.H. Ardinger, R.A. Pagon, et al.). Seattle, WA: University of Washington.

21. A Brief Guide to Genomics. https://www.genome.gov/18016863/a-brief-guide-to-genomics/ (accessed 26 July 2021).

22. Stevenson, R.E., Allanson, J.G., Everman, D.B., and Solomon, B.D. (2016). *Human Malformations and Related Anomalies*. Oxford; New York: Oxford University Press.

23. Cummings, B.B., Marshall, J.L., Tukiainen, T., Lek, M., Donkervoort, S., Foley, A.R., Bolduc, V., Waddell, L.B., Sandaradura, S.A., O'Grady, G.L., et al. (2017). Improving

genetic diagnosis in Mendelian disease with transcriptome sequencing. Sci. Transl. Med. 9(386):eaal5209. doi: https://doi.org/10.1126/scitranslmed.aal5209.

24. Fresard, L., Smail, C., Ferraro, N.M. et al. (2019). Identification of rare-disease genes using blood transcriptome sequencing and large control cohorts. *Nat. Med.* 25: 911–919.

25. Schmerler, S. and Wessel, G.M. (2011). Polar bodies – more a lack of understanding than a lack of respect. *Mol. Reprod. Dev.* 78: 3–8.

26. MedlinePlus Genetics. https://medlineplus.gov/genetics/ (accessed 26 July 2021).

27. Richards, S., Aziz, N., Bale, S. et al. (2015). Standards and guidelines for the interpretation of sequence variants: a joint consensus recommendation of the American College of Medical Genetics and Genomics and the Association for Molecular Pathology. *Genet. Med.* 17: 405–424.

28. Jarvik, G.P. and Evans, J.P. (2017). Mastering genomic terminology. *Genet. Med.* 19: 491–492.

29. den Dunnen, J.T. (2016). Sequence variant descriptions: HGVS nomenclature and mutalyzer. *Curr. Protoc. Hum. Genet.* 90: 7 13 11–7 13 19.

30. Orioli, I.M., Amar, E., Arteaga-Vazquez, J. et al. (2011). Sirenomelia: an epidemiologic study in a large dataset from the International Clearinghouse of Birth Defects Surveillance and Research, and literature review. *Am. J. Med. Genet. C Semin. Med. Genet.* 157C: 358–373.

31. Boer, L.L., Morava, E., Klein, W.M. et al. (2017). Sirenomelia: a multi-systemic polytopic field defect with ongoing controversies. *Birth Defects Res.* 109: 791–804.

32. Biesecker, L.G. and Spinner, N.B. (2013). A genomic view of mosaicism and human disease. *Nat. Rev. Genet.* 14: 307–320.

33. Stosser, M.B., Lindy, A.S., Butler, E. et al. (2018). High frequency of mosaic pathogenic variants in genes causing epilepsy-related neurodevelopmental disorders. *Genet. Med.* 20: 403–410.

34. McClellan, J. and King, M.C. (2010). Genetic heterogeneity in human disease. *Cell* 141: 210–217.

35. Jordan, E. and Hershberger, R.E. (2021). Considering complexity in the genetic evaluation of dilated cardiomyopathy. *Heart* 107: 106–112.

36. ENCODE Project Consortium (2012). An integrated encyclopedia of DNA elements in the human genome. *Nature* 489: 57–74.

37. Watrin, F., Manent, J.B., Cardoso, C., and Represa, A. (2015). Causes and consequences of gray matter heterotopia. *CNS Neurosci. Ther.* 21: 112–122.

38. Romero, D.M., Bahi-Buisson, N., and Francis, F. (2018). Genetics and mechanisms leading to human cortical malformations. *Semin. Cell Dev. Biol.* 76: 33–75.

39. Ho, R. and Hegele, R.A. (2019). Complex effects of laminopathy mutations on nuclear structure and function. *Clin. Genet.* 95: 199–209.

40. Stephens, P.J., Greenman, C.D., Fu, B. et al. (2011). Massive genomic rearrangement acquired in a single catastrophic event during cancer development. *Cell* 144: 27–40.

41. Zhang, C.Z., Spektor, A., Cornils, H. et al. (2015). Chromothripsis from DNA damage in micronuclei. *Nature* 522: 179–184.

42. Cortes-Ciriano, I., Lee, J.J., Xi, R. et al. (2020). Comprehensive analysis of chromothripsis in 2,658 human cancers using whole-genome sequencing. *Nat. Genet.* 52: 331–341.

43. Scitable by Nature Education. https://www.nature.com/scitable/definition/exon-exons-270/ (accessed 26 July 2021).

44. Freyer, C., Cree, L.M., Mourier, A. et al. (2012). Variation in germline mtDNA heteroplasmy is determined prenatally but modified during subsequent transmission. *Nat. Genet.* 44: 1282–1285.

45. Stewart, J.B. and Chinnery, P.F. (2015). The dynamics of mitochondrial DNA heteroplasmy: implications for human health and disease. *Nat. Rev. Genet.* 16: 530–542.

46. Yoneda, Y., Haginoya, K., Kato, M. et al. (2013). Phenotypic spectrum of COL4A1 mutations: porencephaly to schizencephaly. *Ann. Neurol.* 73: 48–57.

47. Del Giudice, E., Macca, M., Imperati, F. et al. (2014). CNS involvement in OFD1 syndrome: a clinical, molecular, and neuroimaging study. *Orphanet J. Rare Dis.* 9: 74.

48. National Human Genome Research Institute Talking Glossary of Genetic Terms. https://www.genome.gov/genetics-glossary/Centromere (accessed 26 July 2021).

49. National Human Genome Research Institute Talking Glossary of Genetic Terms. https://www.genome.gov/genetics-glossary/histone (accessed 26 July 2021).

50. Watson, J.D. and Crick, F.H. (1953). Molecular structure of nucleic acids; a structure for deoxyribose nucleic acid. *Nature* 171: 737–738.

51. Mitsui, Y., Langridge, R., Shortle, B.E. et al. (1970). Physical and enzymatic studies on poly d(I-C)-poly d(I-C), an unusual double-helical DNA. *Nature* 228: 1166–1169.

52. Wang, J.C. (1979). Helical repeat of DNA in solution. *Proc. Natl Acad. Sci. USA* 76: 200–203.

53. National Human Genome Research Institute Talking Glossary of Genetic Terms. https://www.genome.gov/genetics-glossary/Autosome (accessed 26 July 2021).

54. Chiu, C.Y. and Miller, S.A. (2019). Clinical metagenomics. *Nat. Rev. Genet.* 20: 341–355.

55. Steitz, T.A. (2008). A structural understanding of the dynamic ribosome machine. *Nat. Rev. Mol. Cell Biol.* 9: 242–253.

56. National Human Genome Research Institute Talking Glossary of Genetic Terms. https://www.genome.gov/genetics-glossary/Ribosome (accessed 26 July 2021).

57. Doudna, J.A. and Charpentier, E. (2014). Genome editing. The new frontier of genome engineering with CRISPR-Cas9. *Science* 346: 1258096.

58. Adli, M. (2018). The CRISPR tool kit for genome editing and beyond. *Nat. Commun.* 9: 1911.

59. Andersson, R. and Sandelin, A. (2020). Determinants of enhancer and promoter activities of regulatory elements. *Nat. Rev. Genet.* 21: 71–87.

60. National Human Genome Research Institute Talking Glossary of Genetic Terms. https://www.genome.gov/genetics-glossary/Promoter (accessed 26 July 2021).

61. Avner, P. and Heard, E. (2001). X-chromosome inactivation: counting, choice and initiation. *Nat. Rev. Genet.* 2: 59–67.

62. Galupa, R. and Heard, E. (2018). X-chromosome inactivation: a crossroads between chromosome architecture and gene regulation. *Annu. Rev. Genet.* 52: 535–566.

63. Dowsett, L., Porras, A.R., Kruszka, P. et al. (2019). Cornelia de Lange syndrome in diverse populations. *Am. J. Med. Genet. A* 179: 150–158.

64. Meyer, M., Kircher, M., Gansauge, M.T. et al. (2012). A high-coverage genome sequence from an archaic Denisovan individual. *Science* 338: 222–226.

65. Hellenthal, G., Busby, G.B.J., Band, G. et al. (2014). A genetic atlas of human admixture history. *Science* 343: 747–751.

66. Rivlin, N., Brosh, R., Oren, M., and Rotter, V. (2011). Mutations in the p53 tumor suppressor gene: important milestones at the various steps of tumorigenesis. *Genes Cancer* 2: 466–474.

67. Schneider, K., Zelley, K., Nichols, K.E., and Garber, J. (1993). Li-Fraumeni syndrome. In: *GeneReviews*® (ed. M.P. Adam, H.H. Ardinger, R.A. Pagon, et al.). Seattle, WA: University of Washington.

68. Nakagome, Y., Matsubara, T., and Fujita, H. (1983). Distribution of break points in human structural rearrangements. *Am. J. Hum. Genet.* 35: 288–300.

69. Tuck-Muller, C.M., Chen, H., Martinez, J.E. et al. (1995). Isodicentric Y chromosome: cytogenetic, molecular and clinical studies and review of the literature. *Hum. Genet.* 96: 119–129.

70. Lusk, L., Vogel-Farley, V., DiStefano, C., and Jeste, S. (1993). Maternal 15q duplication syndrome. In: *GeneReviews*® (ed. M.P. Adam, H.H. Ardinger, R.A. Pagon, et al.). Seattle, WA: University of Washington.

71. Elmore, S. (2007). Apoptosis: a review of programmed cell death. *Toxicol. Pathol.* 35: 495–516.

72. Singh, R., Letai, A., and Sarosiek, K. (2019). Regulation of apoptosis in health and disease: the balancing act of BCL-2 family proteins. *Nat. Rev. Mol. Cell Biol.* 20: 175–193.

73. National Human Genome Research Institute Talking Glossary of Genetic Terms. https://www.genome.gov/genetics-glossary/apoptosis (accessed 26 July 2021).

74. National Human Genome Research Institute Talking Glossary of Genetic Terms. https://www.genome.gov/genetics-glossary/Transfer-RNA (accessed 26 July 2021).

75. Haubold, B. and Wiehe, T. (2006). How repetitive are genomes? *BMC Bioinform.* 7: 541.

76. Hannan, A.J. (2018). Tandem repeats mediating genetic plasticity in health and disease. *Nat. Rev. Genet.* 19: 286–298.

77. Mitra, I., Huang, B., Mousavi, N. et al. (2021). Patterns of de novo tandem repeat mutations and their role in autism. *Nature* 589: 246–250.

78. Staretz-Chacham, O., Lang, T.C., LaMarca, M.E. et al. (2009). Lysosomal storage disorders in the newborn. *Pediatrics* 123: 1191–1207.

79. Lachmann, R.H. (2020). Treating lysosomal storage disorders: what have we learnt? *J. Inherit. Metab. Dis.* 43: 125–132.

80. National Human Genome Research Institute Talking Glossary of Genetic Terms. https://www.genome.gov/genetics-glossary/Lysosome (accessed 26 July 2021).

81. McGuire, A.L. and Majumder, M.A. (2009). Two cheers for GINA? *Genome Med.* 1: 6.

82. Lenartz, A., Scherer, A.M., Uhlmann, W.R. et al. (2021). The persistent lack of knowledge and misunderstanding of the Genetic Information Nondiscrimination Act (GINA) more than a decade after passage. *Genet. Med.* 23: 2471.

83. National Human Genome Research Institute Talking Glossary of Genetic Terms. https://www.genome.gov/about-genomics/policy-issues/Genetic-Discrimination (accessed 26 July 2021).

84. Song, X., Haghighi, A., Iliuta, I.A., and Pei, Y. (2017). Molecular diagnosis of autosomal dominant polycystic kidney disease. *Expert. Rev. Mol. Diagn.* 17: 885–895.

85. National Human Genome Research Institute Talking Glossary of Genetic Terms. https://www.genome.gov/genetics-glossary/Pseudogene (accessed 26 July 2021).

86. Hassold, T. and Hunt, P. (2001). To err (meiotically) is human: the genesis of human aneuploidy. *Nat. Rev. Genet.* 2: 280–291.

Physical Examination

2

2.1. An infant is noted to have physical examination findings consistent with ulnar deficiency. Based on these findings, which of the following syndromes is the infant most likely to have?

A. CHARGE syndrome

B. Cornelia de Lange syndrome

C. Kabuki syndrome

D. Pallister-Hall syndrome

2.2. A patient undergoing examination has an occipito-frontal head circumference (OFC) at least two standard deviations below the mean (as adjusted for factors such as age and sex). What term describes this finding?

A. Brachycephaly

B. Dolicocephaly

C. Macrocephaly

D. Microcephaly

2.3. What condition is most likely pictured in the photo below?

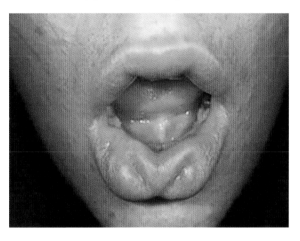

Source: National Human Genome Research Institute: Elements of Morphology: Human Malformation Terminology [1].

A. Achondroplasia

B. Pfeiffer syndrome

C. Stickler syndrome

D. Van der Woude syndrome

2.4. Which physical examination finding is NOT characteristic of fetal alcohol syndrome?

A. Microcephaly

B. Frontal bossing

C. Short palpebral fissures

D. Smooth philtrum

Medical Genetics and Genomics: Questions for Board Review, First Edition. Benjamin D. Solomon.
© 2023 John Wiley & Sons Ltd. Published 2023 by John Wiley & Sons Ltd.

2.5. Genetics is consulted because an infant is noted to have "puffy hands and feet." Based on this information, what genetic condition would likely be suspected?

A. Alport syndrome
C. Joubert syndrome
B. Fragile X syndrome
D. Turner syndrome

2.6. An infant was slightly premature and is being taken care of in the NICU; on rounds, the team notes "puffiness" under the eyes, and that the calcium level has been high on routine blood chemistries. What genetic condition might be suspected based on this?

A. 22q11.2 deletion syndrome
C. Marfan syndrome
B. Homocystinuria
D. Williams syndrome

2.7. A parent has the dental finding shown in the photo below. What associated condition might occur in this person's child?

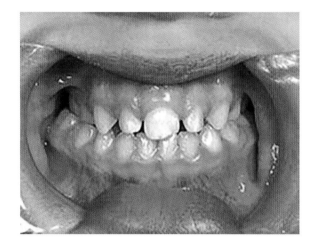

Source: National Human Genome Research Institute: Elements of Morphology: Human Malformation Terminology [1].

A. Lissencephaly
C. Brachycephaly
B. Holoprosencephaly
D. Trigonocephaly

2.8. A child has craniosynostosis and is also noted to have syndactyly. Which craniosynostosis syndrome is most likely?

A. Apert syndrome
C. Crouzon syndrome
B. Beare-Stevenson
D. Pfeiffer syndrome

2.9. A patient has Moebius sequence. On exam, one might expect to see signs of bilateral congenital paralysis of which cranial nerves?

A. 1 and 2
C. 6 and 7
B. 5 and 10
D. All cranial nerves

2.10. An infant with Y-shaped 2–3 toe syndactyly might be suspected to have what condition?

A. Adams-Oliver syndrome
C. Smith-Lemli-Opitz syndrome
B. Silver-Russell syndrome
D. Trisomy 18

2.11. What is the technical term for the appearance of the eyebrows in the photo shown below?

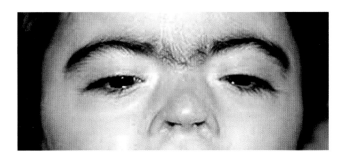

Source: Hall et al. [2].

A. Coloboma   C. Ptosis

B. Epicanthus   D. Synophrys

2.12. On physical exam, a child is noted to have unilateral leukocoria (the pupillary reflex appears white during the eye exam). Which condition might be suspected?

A. Macular degeneration   C. Retinoblastoma

B. Retinitis pigmentosa   D. Tay-Sachs disease

2.13. What "biochemical" condition can have features on physical examination that resemble some of those seen in people with Marfan syndrome?

A. Galactosemia   C. Maple syrup urine disease

B. Homocystinuria   D. Phenylketonuria

2.14. Which term refers to lateral curvature of a digit, as in the fifth finger in the image shown below?

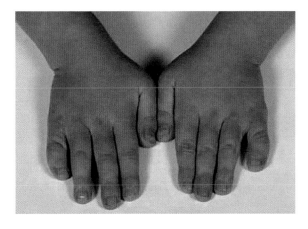

Source: Biesecker et al. [3].

A. Brachydactyly   C. Clinodactyly

B. Camptodactyly   D. Polydactyly

2.15. What physical examination finding would most likely be observed in a person with Wilson disease?

A. Coloboma

B. Lisch nodules

C. Kayser-Fleischer rings

D. Xanthelasma

2.16. An infant has multiple congenital contractures affecting more than one different area of the body. Which term describes this finding?

A. Arthritis

B. Arthrogryposis

C. Hypochondrogenesis

D. Talipes equinovarus

2.17. On examination, an infant has the findings shown in the image below. Which condition might be considered?

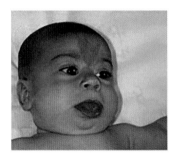

Source: Mussa et al. [4].

A. Beckwith-Wiedemann syndrome

B. Down syndrome

C. Prader-Willi syndrome

D. Trisomy 18

2.18. What condition includes physical examination findings including aplasia cutis congenita of the scalp and terminal transverse limb defects?

A. Adams-Oliver syndrome

B. Baller-Gerold syndrome

C. Chediak-Higashi syndrome

D. Donnai-Barrow syndrome

2.19. Which facial feature affecting the nose would likely be observed in a person with Rubinstein-Taybi syndrome?

A. Absent nose

B. Anteverted nares

C. Bifid nasal tip

D. Low hanging columella

2.20. People with Robin (Pierre-Robin) sequence frequently have which finding noted on physical examination?

A. Amelia

B. Cleft palate

C. Mirror movements

D. Omphalocele

2.21. Which part of the body is most commonly affected by amniotic bands?

A. Abdomen

B. Face

C. Heart

D. Limbs

2.22. A "two-vessel cord," which may be identified during the immediate neonatal exam or prenatally, typically refers to what arrangement for the blood vessels in the umbilical cord?

A. 1 artery, 1 vein

B. 2 arteries

C. 2 arteries, 1 vein

D. 2 veins

2.23. On examination, a girl is noted to have coarse facial features, hepatosplenomegaly, short stature, corneal clouding, developmental delay and limited range of motion of the joints. Which condition is most likely?

A. Hunter syndrome   C. Morquio syndrome
B. Hurler syndrome   D. Rett syndrome

2.24. An infant has polydactyly and a midline cleft lip. What trisomy would be most likely?

A. Trisomy 1   C. Trisomy 18
B. Trisomy 13   D. Trisomy 21

2.25. A patient has a family history of sudden death. The patient's hands look like the image shown below. What condition is most likely?

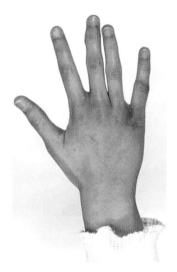

Source: Biesecker et al. [3].

A. Fanconi anemia   C. Marfan syndrome
B. Holt-Oram syndrome   D. Short QT syndrome

2.26. On neurological exam, a patient is noted to have involuntary movements affecting the hands on one side of the body, which copy intentional movements on the other side. What is the term for this?

A. Dystonia   C. Seizures
B. Mirror movements   D. Tics

2.27. A toddler with a history of developmental delay and seizures is noted to have hypopigmented streaks following the lines of Blaschko. What condition might be considered as likely?

A. Hypomelanosis of Ito   C. Neurofibromatosis type 2
B. Klippel-Trenaunay syndrome   D. McCune-Albright syndrome

2.28. What eye finding might be noted in a person with Tay-Sachs disease?

A. Anophthalmia

B. Cherry-red spot

C. Coloboma

D. Lisch nodules

2.29. An infant boy is noted to have a congenital anomaly in which there is ventral and proximal displacement of the urethral meatus from the tip of the glans penis. Which term best describes this finding?

A. Epispadias

B. Hydrocele

C. Hypospadias

D. Müllerian aplasia

2.30. Which feature on physical examination may be expected to be observed in individuals with Russell-Silver syndrome?

A. Coarse features

B. Macrosomia

C. Tall stature

D. Triangular facies

2.31. Which "scoring system" or scale is used on physical examination to assess joint hypermobility, as in the assessment of a person with possible Ehlers-Danlos syndrome?

A. Amsterdam

B. Beighton

C. Ghent

D. Vanderbilt

2.32. A neonate has an abdominal wall defect lateral to the umbilicus; there is no protective membrane around the herniated abdominal contents. What type of congenital anomaly is this?

A. Gastroschisis

B. Hydrocele

C. Omphalocele

D. Situs inversus

2.33. On examination, a 10-year-old child and her father are found to have open anterior fontanelles, as well as dental anomalies. In these patients, what other part of the body would be the most likely to be found to be affected?

A. Clavicles

B. Heart

C. Kidneys

D. Spleen

2.34. An infant has an anteriorly attached lingual frenulum, and limited tongue mobility, referred to as a "tongue tie" by the parents. What is the term for this finding?

A. Ankyloglossia

B. Glossoptosis

C. Oligodontia

D. Macroglossia

2.35. Which of the following conditions frequently includes the exam finding of microcephaly (versus macrocephaly)?

A. Pallister-Hall syndrome

B. Seckel syndrome

C. Simpson-Golabi-Behmel syndrome

D. Sotos syndrome

2.36. An individual has been diagnosed with primary trimethylaminuria. Which of the following best describes the odor associated with this condition?

A. Fishy

B. Musty

C. Sweaty socks

D. Sugary/sweet

2.37. An infant is noticed to have a high-pitched cry that sounds like a cat crying. What genetic change is most likely to account for this?
A. 1p36 deletion
B. 5p-
C. Monosomy X
D. Tetraploidy

2.38. An adult, who is new to a medical practice, comes in for her routine check-up. She has the findings shown in the image below. What condition would likely be suspected?

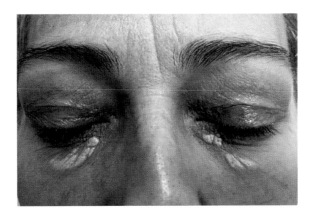

Source: Baroni [5].
A. Acute intermittent porphyria
B. Familial hypercholesterolemia
C. Neurofibromatosis type 1
D. Wilson disease

2.39. A patient is initially seen by a primary care doctor because of neck pain. They are referred to genetics when the doctor notices they have a short neck with limited mobility; X-rays show evidence of cervical vertebral fusion. Which condition often involves these findings?
A. CHARGE syndrome
B. Cleidocranial dysostosis
C. Hypochondrogenesis
D. Klippel-Feil syndrome

2.40. Based on history and physical examination, an adolescent is noted to have features of a heritable connective tissue disorder. Which of the following syndromes is NOT traditionally considered a heritable connective tissue disorder?
A. Ehlers-Danlos syndrome
B. Klinefelter syndrome
C. Loeys-Dietz syndrome
D. Marfan syndrome

2.41. A newborn is small for gestational age and has a structural cardiac anomaly. On examination, a prominent occiput, short palpebral fissures, low-set ears, micrognathia, and clenched hands are noted. Which condition is most likely?
A. Trisomy 13
B. Trisomy 18
C. Trisomy 21
D. Turner syndrome

2.42. On examination, a patient is noted to have an opacity affecting the crystalline lens of the eye. What is the best term for this finding?

A. Cataract
C. Coloboma

B. Cherry-red spot
D. Cryptophthalmos

2.43. A child is brought to see a geneticist due to distinctive facial features and hypertrophic cardiomyopathy. On exam, the skin appears as shown. What is the most likely condition?

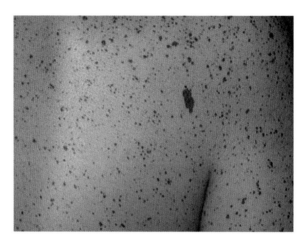

Source: Rodríguez-Bujaldón et al. [6].

A. Incontinentia pigmenti
C. Tuberous sclerosis

B. Noonan syndrome with multiple lentigines
D. Xeroderma pigmentosum

2.44. A patient has been diagnosed with Gilbert syndrome. What clinical feature would be most likely to be noticed on examination?

A. Epidermolysis
C. Strabismus

B. Hyperbilirubinemia
D. Telangiectasias

2.45. A child with hearing loss is noted to have a depigmented hair patch, and heterochromia iridis (the eyes are different colors). What condition might be suspected?

A. Alport syndrome
C. Waardenburg syndrome

B. Treacher-Collins syndrome
D. Walker-Warburg syndrome

2.46. Which condition does NOT frequently involve early overgrowth?

A. Beckwith-Wiedemann syndrome
C. Sotos syndrome

B. Seckel syndrome
D. Weaver syndrome

2.47. A person has wide spacing between the inner canthi but the interpupillary distance is normal. What is the best way to describe this?

A. Hypotelorism
C. Proptosis

B. Hypertelorism
D. Telecanthus

2.48. A patient has been diagnosed with Albright hereditary osteodystrophy. On physical examination, what hand finding would most likely be noticed regarding the fourth and fifth digits?

A. Arachnodactyly
B. Brachydactyly
C. Oligodactyly
D. Syndactyly

2.49. A child has been diagnosed with Congenital generalized lipodystrophy (Berardinelli-Seip congenital lipodystrophy). Which finding on physical examination would be most typical of this condition?

A. Alopecia
B. Lipoatrophy
C. Obesity
D. Polydactyly

2.50. On examination, a patient is noted to have repetitive, involuntary eye movements. What is the best description for this finding?

A. Coloboma
B. Mydriasis
C. Nystagmus
D. Retinitis pigmentosa

2.51. What finding does the following image depict?

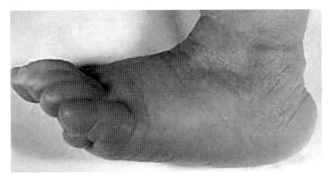

Source: Biesecker et al. [3].

A. Camptodactyly
B. Pes cavus
C. Rocker bottom foot
D. Sandal gap

2.52. A one-year-old child with a suspected genetic condition is examined. By this age, the anterior fontanel will be closed in about what percent of infants?

A. 1%
B. 20%
C. 40%
D. 90%

2.53. Which condition can involve, among findings affecting other organ systems, skin findings such as hypomelanotic macules (including "ash leaf spots"), Shagreen patches, facial angiofibromas, and "confetti" skin lesions?

A. Hypomelanosis of Ito
B. Neurofibromatosis type 1
C. Noonan syndrome
D. Tuberous sclerosis complex

2.54. Genetics is consulted because a young patient has a hand malformation and ipsilateral pectoralis major hypoplasia. Which term refers to the findings seen in this patient?

A. Klippel-Feil anomaly
B. Pectus carinatum
C. Poland anomaly
D. Sprengel anomaly

2.55. A person with a genetic condition is noted to have small, white-grayish spots around the periphery of the iris (see example in the image below). What condition is most likely?

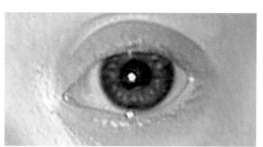

Source: Wikimedia Commons [7]

A. Down syndrome

B. Neurofibromatosis type 1

C. Waardenburg syndrome

D. Williams syndrome

Answers

2.1. B	2.15. C	2.29. C	2.43. B
2.2. D	2.16. B	2.30. D	2.44. B
2.3. D	2.17. A	2.31. B	2.45. C
2.4. B	2.18. A	2.32. A	2.46. B
2.5. D	2.19. D	2.33. A	2.47. D
2.6. D	2.20. B	2.34. A	2.48. B
2.7. B	2.21. D	2.35. B	2.49. B
2.8. A	2.22. A	2.36. A	2.50. C
2.9. C	2.23. B	2.37. B	2.51. C
2.10. C	2.24. B	2.38. B	2.52. C
2.11. D	2.25. C	2.39. D	2.53. D
2.12. C	2.26. B	2.40. B	2.54. C
2.13. B	2.27. A	2.41. B	2.55. A
2.14. C	2.28. B	2.42. A	

Commentary

2.1. Cornelia de Lange syndrome

Cornelia de Lange syndrome (CdLS) is a genetic condition that can include distinctive craniofacial features (including microbrachycephaly, synophrys, highly arched eyebrows, long and thick eyelashes, and short nose with anteverted nares), hirsutism, growth impairment, intellectual disability, and a range of upper limb deficits primarily involving the ulnar structures, as well as other anomalies. Upper limb anomalies can range from mild fifth digit hypoplasia to complete forearm absence. CdLS can be caused by pathogenic variants in *NIPBL* (accounting for ~60% of CdLS), *RAD21*, *SMC3*, *HDAC8*, and *SMC1A*; inheritance can be autosomal dominant (usually de novo) or X-linked.

Reference(s): Deardorff et al. [8]; Mehta et al. [9]; Jones et al. [10].

2.2. Microcephaly

Microcephaly is defined as an occipito-frontal head circumference (OFC) at least two standard deviations smaller than the mean, as adjusted for factors such as age (including gestational age, where appropriate) and sex. Microcephaly can be congenital (primary) or acquired (secondary). Microcephaly can be caused by genetic or nongenetic factors and can occur in an isolated or syndromic fashion. Many hundreds of genes have been implicated in causes of microcephaly, and up to about half of individuals with microcephaly have been reported to have a genetic cause.

Reference(s): Ashwal et al. [11]; Duerinckx and Abramowicz [12].

2.3. Van der Woude syndrome

Van der Woude syndrome (VWS) is a dominant condition caused by pathogenic variants in the gene *IRF6*. Common features include congenital, often bilateral, lower lip pits, cleft lip, cleft palate, and submucous cleft palate. Pathogenic variants in *IRF6* can cause a range of phenotypes – even within a single family – including isolated cleft lip and palate, VWS, and Popliteal pterygium syndrome (PPS). PPS can include findings seen in VWS, as well as additional anomalies such as popliteal pterygia (webbing of the skin from the ischial tuberosities to the heels), genitourinary anomalies, ankyloblepharon (eyelid synechiae), pyramidal fold of skin overlying the nail of the hallux, and intraoral adhesions.

Reference(s): Busche et al. [13]; Schutte et al. [14].

2.4. Frontal bossing

Fetal alcohol syndrome is due to maternal alcohol consumption during pregnancy. The type and severity of effects are influenced by the timing and amount of alcohol consumption, as well as other incompletely understood factors. The main features include prenatal and postnatal growth restriction, neurologic and neurobehavioral sequelae, and craniofacial and other physical manifestations. Physical examination features can include microcephaly, as well as short palpebral fissures, smooth philtrum, and narrow vermilion border of the upper lip (thin upper lip). Other craniofacial features can include findings such as flat midface, ptosis, epicanthal folds, short nose, and ears with a "railroad" track appearance. Additional physical examination features can include hirsutism, fifth finger clinodactyly, camptodactyly, and "hockey stick" pattern of the palmar creases. Individuals may also have other features such as cardiac anomalies.

Reference(s): Wattendorf and Muenke [15]; Del Campo and Jones [16]; Jones et al. [10].

2.5. Turner syndrome

Clinical manifestations of Turner syndrome can include findings related to congenital lymphedema (which can include "puffy hands and feet" and redundant nuchal skin), short stature, and gonadal dysgenesis. Turner syndrome occurs in about 1 in 2500 live-born female infants and results from the absence of all or part of the X chromosome. In up to 33% of individuals, the condition is identified in infancy due to features such as puffy hands and feet or redundant nuchal skin. Additional features that may manifest or be identified at different ages can include congenital heart anomalies (bicuspid aortic valve, coarctation of the aorta, and other left-sided heart anomalies), short stature, and amenorrhea, as well as other findings.

Reference(s): Sybert and McCauley [17]; Jones et al. [18].

2.6. Williams syndrome

Williams syndrome occurs due to heterozygous deletion of chromosome 7q11.23. The condition affects multiple organ systems, and often includes a distinctive facial appearance that evolves as the person ages (in infancy this can include periorbital fullness, as well as other findings), cardiovascular anomalies (e.g., supravalvar aortic stenosis), endocrine disorders (including neonatal hypercalcemia and hypercalciuria), and other features.

Reference(s): Strømme et al. [19]; Morris et al. [20].

2.7. Holoprosencephaly

The photo shows a single maxillary central incisor (SMCI). This finding may be seen in individuals with "microform" holoprosencephaly (HPE). Microform HPE typically involves subtle midline craniofacial manifestations, such as hypotelorism (close-set eyes) and SMCI, without clear neuroanatomic anomalies. Microform HPE may be caused by pathogenic variants in genes such as *SHH* or *SIX3*. These variants are inherited in an autosomal dominant manner, and there is highly variable expressivity and incomplete penetrance. If affected, children who inherit these variants may have microform HPE or frank HPE. HPE involves midline brain anomalies due to failed or incomplete separation of the developing forebrain. The severity ranges from prenatal lethality to severe neurocognitive dysfunction. HPE is usually accompanied by midline craniofacial findings, as well as other features such as pituitary insufficiency (especially diabetes insipidus) and seizures. There are many causes of HPE in addition to pathogenic variants in these genes.

Reference(s): Dubourg et al. [21]; Solomon et al. [22].

2.8. Apert syndrome

Apert syndrome, which is caused by heterozygous pathogenic variants in *FGFR2*, includes craniosynostosis and can include soft tissue or bony syndactyly of the fingers and toes. In addition to craniosynostosis and limb findings, patients with Apert syndrome can also have developmental delay/intellectual disability and additional skeletal and other anomalies. Pathogenic variants in *FGFR2* can cause other craniosynostosis syndromes, as well as other disorders.

Reference(s): Agochukwu et al. [23]; Wenger et al. [24].

2.9. 6 and 7

Moebius sequence (MS) refers to congenital paralysis of the sixth and seventh cranial nerves, the abducens, and facial nerves. This paralysis is usually bilateral and manifests with lack of both facial expressions/movement and horizontal eye movement. Feeding is often impacted. The condition may be accompanied by additional anomalies affecting the face or other parts of the body. MS is typically sporadic; the causes remain overall unclear, though a variety and nongenetic factors have been implicated.

Reference(s): Kjeldgaard Pedersen et al. [25]; Jones et al. [18].

2.10. Smith-Lemli Opitz syndrome

Smith-Lemli-Opitz syndrome (SLOS) is an autosomal recessive cholesterol metabolism disorder due to pathogenic variants in the gene *DHCR7*. Clinical manifestations can include microcephaly, intellectual disability, decreased growth, characteristic facial features and other malformations including cleft palate, congenital heart defects, underdeveloped external genitalia in males, postaxial polydactyly, and 2-3 toe syndactyly. Diagnosis can be confirmed through molecular testing and through elevated 7-dehydrocholesterol levels, often (though not always) with low total cholesterol.

Reference(s): Porter [26]; Nowaczyk and Wassif [27].

2.11. Synophrys

Synophrys refers to the meeting of the medial eyebrows in the midline. Synophrys may be seen in a number of different genetic conditions, including Cornelia de Lange syndrome, several chromosomal/cytogenomic conditions, Smith-Magenis syndrome, and others.

Reference(s): Jones et al. [18].

2.12. Retinoblastoma

Retinoblastoma, a malignant retinal tumor, typically occurs in children before five years of age. The condition is related to variants in the gene *RB1*. Signs of retinoblastoma may include leukocoria (an abnormally pupillary reflex with a white appearance to the pupil on eye examination), strabismus, and decreased vision. Some affected individuals may have other medical or family history suggesting hereditary retinoblastoma.

Reference(s): Lohmann and Gallie [28].

2.13. Homocystinuria

Homocystinuria due to cystathionine β-synthase deficiency can involve manifestations affecting different body systems, including the ophthalmologic (severe myopia, ectopia lentis), skeletal (tall stature with long limbs, scoliosis, pectus excavatum), vascular (thromboembolism), and central nervous (intellectual disability) systems. Marfan syndrome and homocystinuria's shared features can include a similar thin and tall body habitus, arachnodactyly, and predisposition for certain ophthalmologic manifestations (myopia, ectopia lentis).

Reference(s): Summers et al. [29]; Sacharow et al. [30].

2.14. Clinodactyly

Clinodactyly refers to a digit that is laterally curved (in the plane of the palm). The photo shown in the question depicts fifth finger ("pinky") clinodactyly. Clinodactyly, which is often due to an abnormally shaped middle phalanx, involves the phalanges rather than deviation at the more proximal joints. Clinodactyly can affect any digit and can be in either direction, but radial deviation of the fifth finger is the most common type. Many genetic conditions can have fifth finger clinodactyly.

Reference(s): Jones et al. [18].

2.15. Kayser-Fleischer rings

Wilson disease, caused by biallelic pathogenic variants in *ATP7B*, is a copper metabolism disorder that can involve liver disease, neurologic, and psychiatric manifestations. The condition can be highly variable, with signs and symptoms arising from early childhood through late adulthood. Kayser-Fleischer rings, which refer to brown-colored peripheral corneal copper deposits, have been reported in about half of patients with Wilson disease and liver disease and about 90% of those with neurologic or psychiatric manifestations. Wilson disease can be diagnosed through observation of clinical/biochemical features and testing (including Kayser-Fleischer rings, low serum copper and ceruloplasmin concentrations, high urinary copper excretion) and/or molecular testing. Treatment is available through copper-chelating agents or zinc, but liver transplantation may be necessary.

Reference(s:) Bandmann et al. [31]; Weiss [32].

2.16. Arthrogryposis

Arthrogryposis refers to the presence of congenital contractures that affect multiple different areas of the body. Arthrogryposis is seen in about 1 in 3000 live births and may occur as a feature in hundreds of different conditions. There are multiple types and subtypes of the disorder, and there are many known genetic and nongenetic causes. One of the important first distinctions in the clinical evaluation is whether a patient has neurologic dysfunction.

Reference(s): Bamshad et al. [33]; Hall and Kiefer [34].

2.17. Beckwith-Wiedemann syndrome

Beckwith-Wiedemann syndrome (BWS) is a multisystem pediatric overgrowth condition that results from abnormal regulation of gene transcription affecting two imprinted domains on chromosome 11p15.5. BWS can sometimes be recognized by clinical manifestations observed in affected infants. Clinical features of BWS can involve macroglossia (the large tongue shown in the image in the question), neonatal hypoglycemia, macrosomia, hemihyperplasia, omphalocele, visceromegaly, adrenocortical cytomegaly, renal abnormalities, and ear creases/pits.

Reference(s): Weksberg et al. [35]; Shuman et al. [36]; Nussbaum et al. [37].

2.18. Adams-Oliver syndrome

Adams-Oliver syndrome includes aplasia cutis congenita of the scalp and terminal transverse limb defects, though other anomalies, such as cardiac malformations, may also be identified. Pathogenic variants in multiple genes can cause Adams-Oliver syndrome, with both dominant and recessively inherited forms described.

Reference(s): Lehman et al. [38]; Hassed et al. [39].

2.19. Low-hanging columella

Rubinstein-Taybi syndrome (RTS) is classically described as including broad and often angulated thumbs and great toes, intellectual disability, short stature, and distinctive facial features. These facial features include downslanted palpebral fissures, low-hanging columella, high palate, "grimacing smile," and talon cusps. RTS is caused by heterozygous pathogenic variants in the genes *CREBBP* and *EP300*, though recent evidence suggests clinical differences depending on the underlying gene involved, with "less classic" presentations described related to *EP300*.

Reference(s): Fergelot et al. [40]; Stevens [41].

2.20. Cleft palate

Robin sequence, or Pierre-Robin sequence, refers to the triad of micrognathia, glossoptosis (obstruction of the posterior pharyngeal space by the tongue), and airway obstruction. Cleft palate occurs in up to 90% of patients with Robin sequence. There are many known genetic conditions that can include Robin sequence as a feature.

Reference(s): Evans et al. [42]; Breugem et al. [43].

Chapter 2

2.21. Limbs

Amniotic band syndrome, sometimes called amnion rupture sequence, refers to strands of ruptured amnion that may attach to and affect parts of the developing fetus, including through secondary effects such as decreased fetal movement. There is a wide range of severity, and virtually any part of the body can be impacted, but the limbs are the most frequently affected. The condition typically occurs sporadically; the overall causes and precise biological underpinnings are unclear.

Reference(s): Jones et al. [18]; Stevenson et al. [44].

2.22. 1 artery, 1 vein

Ordinarily, the umbilical cord contains three vessels: two umbilical arteries and one umbilical vein. The umbilical arteries carry deoxygenated blood from the fetus to the placenta, while the umbilical vein carries oxygenated blood from the placenta to the fetus. A "two-vessel" cord (2VC) typically refers to a cord with a single umbilical artery (SUA) such that the umbilical cord contains one umbilical artery and one umbilical vein. The clinical significance of a SUA appears to depend on or at least be related to any accompanying structural anomalies, which may or may not be present. In addition to SUA, there are also other types of umbilical cord anomalies.

Reference(s): Stevenson et al. [44].

2.23. Hurler syndrome

Mucopolysaccharidosis type I (MPS I) is an autosomal recessive condition caused by bi-allelic pathogenic variants in the *IDUA* gene, which encodes the alpha-L-iduronidase enzyme. Traditionally, MPS I was subdivided into Hurler, Hurler-Scheie, and Scheie syndromes, but evidence has demonstrated that these represent a continuum of disease without clear biochemical or clinical distinctions. More recently, instead of the previous classification schema, MPS I has been described as having severe or attenuated forms. Clinical findings, which vary, often include coarse facial features, inguinal and umbilical hernia, hepatosplenomegaly, skeletal changes (gibbus deformity, limited joint mobility, and other findings), frequent otitis media and other upper respiratory infections, cardiac valvular anomalies affecting heart function, hearing loss, developmental delay, and corneal clouding. Testing results from urinary glycosaminoglycans can help support the diagnosis.

Reference(s): Clarke [45]; Jones et al. [18].

2.24. Trisomy 13

Findings in patients with trisomy 13, sometimes referred to as Patau syndrome, can include midline brain anomalies in the holoprosencephaly spectrum, as well as accompanying midline facial anomalies (e.g., cleft lip/palate), microphthalmia or other ocular anomalies, hearing impairment, capillary hemangiomata, scalp defects, structural cardiac anomalies, genitourinary anomalies, polydactyly, and other limb anomalies. Many other anomalies have also been described.

Reference(s): Pont et al. [46]; Crider et al. [47]; Jones et al. [18].

2.25. Marfan syndrome

Marfan syndrome is a multisystem connective tissue disorder caused by pathogenic variants in *FBN1*. Variants in this gene can also cause other overlapping phenotypes. Marfan syndrome can affect the heart (including aortic dilatation leading to aortic dissection or rupture), eyes (including myopia and ectopia lentis), and musculoskeletal systems (including, as shown in the image, long fingers, formerly termed "arachnodactyly"). Diagnosis is important for management.

Reference(s): Judge and Dietz [48]; Dietz [49]; Pyeritz [50]; National Human Genome Research Institute: Elements of Morphology: Human Malformation Terminology [1].

2.26. Mirror movements

Congenital mirror movements (CMM) describe a condition where movements on one side of the body involuntarily mirror (mimic) movements on the other side. The onset of CMM is in infancy or early childhood, and the condition persists. The distal upper limbs are usually most affected. Pathogenic variants in several different genes have been identified in individuals with CMM.

Reference(s): Bonnet et al. [51]; Méneret et al. [52].

2.27. Hypomelanosis of Ito

Hypomelanosis of Ito (previously sometimes called incontinentia pigmenti achromians) is a rare neurocutaneous disorder involving hypopigmented streaks, whorls, or mottled areas that follow the lines of Blaschko. These skin findings are typically not evident in infancy but may be apparent within the first few months of life. In addition to the skin lesions, multiple other organ systems can be affected, and patients may have neurologic sequelae including developmental delay and seizures. Different causes (and inheritance patterns) have been suggested, but at least some individuals have been identified as having genetic mosaicism, such as for mosaic cytogenomic abnormalities.

Reference(s): Ream [53]; Jones et al. [18].

2.28. Cherry-red spot

Tay-Sachs disease (TSD), caused by hexosaminidase A deficiency, is due to bi-allelic pathogenic variants in the gene *HEXA*. TSD is a neurodegenerative condition that progresses to death in early childhood. Patients often have weakness and loss of motor milestones noted around 3–6 months of life; physical examination may reveal a cherry-red spot in the macula of the eye. The cherry-red spot is present in this (and other disorders) because storage material abnormally accumulates in the retinal layers of the eye but not in the macule, as the macule doesn't contain as many of these retinal layers. In other words, the cherry-red spot represents a relative absence of the build-up of storage material. Cherry red spots may also be seen in other disorders, such as Niemann-Pick type A.

Reference(s): McGovern et al. [54]; Chen et al. [55]; Toro et al. [56].

2.29. Hypospadias

Hypospadias refers to a type of congenital anomaly where the urethral meatus is displaced ventrally and proximally. In less technical terms, this means that the opening of the penis would occur on the "underside" of the penis and closer to the body. Hypospadias occurs in about 1 in 250 births. There are different types and severities. Overall, the causes remain incompletely understood. Hypospadias can occur in an isolated context or as part of a syndrome with other features.

Reference(s): Macedo et al. [57]; Stevenson et al. [44].

2.30. Triangular facies

Russell-Silver syndrome (sometimes called Silver-Russell syndrome) often includes intrauterine growth restriction (IUGR), postnatal growth deficiency, body asymmetry, distinctive features on physical examination including relative macrocephaly and triangular facies, and risk of developmental delay and learning disabilities. A genetic cause can be found in more than half of affected people; the most common causes identified are loss of chromosome 11p15 methylation and maternal uniparental disomy for chromosome 7.

Reference(s): Eggermann [58]; Wakeling et al. [59]; Saal et al. [60].

2.31. Beighton

Joint hypermobility can be a feature in certain conditions, including "connective tissue disorders" like Ehlers-Danlos syndrome. Joint hypermobility may be assessed using the Beighton scale, which examines the mobility of the fifth fingers, thumbs, elbows, knees, and spine. As an example of how the Beighton score can help diagnostically, generalized joint hypermobility as assessed by the Beighton scale is considered a major diagnostic criteria for classic Ehlers-Danlos syndrome.

Reference(s): Malfait et al. [61]; Malfait et al. [62].

2.32. Gastroschisis

Gastroschisis refers to an abdominal wall defect (occurring lateral to the umbilicus) with herniation of the abdominal wall contents without any protective membrane. Gastroschisis occurs in about 1 in 2000–5000 births and is often detected prenatally. About 10% of affected patients have other anomalies. The causes remain largely unknown, including related to potentially contributory genetic changes.

Reference(s): Hunter and Soothill [63]; Feldkamp et al. [64]; Stevenson et al. [44].

2.33. Clavicles

Cleidocranial dysplasia (also called cleidocranial dysostosis) is an autosomal dominant skeletal disorder caused by pathogenic variants in *RUNX2*; many cases occur de novo. Individuals may have open fontanelles, aplasia or hypoplasia of the clavicles, and dental anomalies. Individuals may also have features such as relatively short stature, other skeletal anomalies, hand anomalies, frequent ear and sinus infections, and upper-airway obstruction.

Reference(s): Cooper et al. [65]; Dinçsoy et al. [66]; Machol et al. [67].

2.34. Anklyoglossia

Ankyloglossia refers to a short or anteriorly attached lingual frenulum, associated with limited tongue mobility. Ankyloglossia can range in severity, from fusion of the tongue to the floor of the mouth to a short frenulum or a frenulum attached more anteriorly than usual, which may be referred to as a "tongue tie."

Reference(s): National Human Genome Research Institute: Elements of Morphology: Human Malformation Terminology [1].

2.35. Seckel syndrome

Macrocephaly is defined as an occipitofrontal circumference (OFC) that is greater than the 98th centile for age. There are many potential underlying causes of macrocephaly, which may occur in a syndromic or nonsyndromic context. Multiple syndromes may frequently include macrocephaly as a features, including Pallister-Hall, Simpson-Golabi-Behmel, and Sotos syndromes, as well as others. Seckel syndrome frequently includes microcephaly, which is defined as an OFC equal to or less than −2 SD below the mean while accounting for sex, age, and ethnicity.

Reference(s): Verloes et al. [68]; Jones et al. [18].

2.36. Fishy

Primary trimethylaminuria is an autosomal recessive biochemical condition caused by bi-allelic pathogenic variants in *FMO3*. The condition involves a fishy odor, which is due to excess excretion of trimethylamine in the urine, breath, sweat, and reproductive fluids. Other inborn errors of metabolism/biochemical conditions may involve other distinct odors (as well as other manifestations).

Reference(s): Mace et al. [69]; Rizzo and Roth [70]; Burton [71]; Phillips and Shephard [72].

2.37. 5p-

5p- syndrome, which results from deletions affecting the short arm of chromosome 5 (5p), is sometimes referred to as Cri du Chat syndrome (CdCS). Frequent clinical features include a high-pitched cry said to sound like the cry of a cat, as well as microcephaly, and distinctive features on physical examination (e.g., broad nasal bridge, epicanthal folds, and micrognathia), growth restriction, and neurocognitive sequelae. Additional features affecting other organ systems may also be present.

Reference(s): Cerruti Mainardi [73]; Nguyen et al. [74].

2.38. Familial hypercholesterolemia

The image accompanying the question shows xanthomas, which are patches of cholesterol build-up, and which frequently occur near the eyelids and on the tendons of the limbs, such as the Achilles tendon. Xanthomas can occur in Familial hypercholesterolemia (FH), a genetic condition that can be due to variants in a number of genes. Another physical examination finding in this condition can be a corneal arcus, which is a ring in the corneal margin. Other features of the condition include high LDL and total cholesterol and signs and symptoms of premature atherosclerosis. Similar findings to those shown in the image can also be seen in Erdheim-Chester disease (ECD).

Reference(s): Bell et al. [75]; Abul-Husn et al. [76]; Goyal et al. [77]; Kobic et al. [78].

2.39. Klippel-Feil syndrome

Klippel-Feil syndrome involves fusion of the cervical vertebrae, which can be accompanied by other anomalies. This can result in physical sequelae, such as a short neck with limited mobility, as well as other manifestations, such as spinal stenosis, neurologic deficits, and neck pain. Different types have been described. Klippel-Feil syndrome is usually sporadic, and the cause is unknown in most individuals, though some genetic causes or susceptibilities have been described.

Reference(s): Klimo et al. [79]; Jones et al. [18].

2.40. Klinefelter syndrome

There are many different heritable connective tissue disorders (HCTDs). In HCTDs, the connective tissue related to multiple organ systems can be affected, including the bones, cardiovascular system, eyes, lungs, joints, and skin. The manifestations can vary between and among different HCTDs, which include Ehlers-Danlos, Loeys-Dietz, and Marfan syndromes, as well as other conditions.

Reference(s): Colombi et al. [80]; Verstraeten et al. [81]; Meester et al. [82]; Jones et al. [18].

2.41. Trisomy 18

Trisomy 18 (occasionally called Edwards syndrome) occurs in about 1 in 5000–8000 live births. Frequent features include intrauterine growth restriction (IUGR) and small for gestational age (SGA) status, structural cardiac malformations, and notable findings on physical examination, such as a prominent occiput, low-set, dysplastic ears, small palpebral fissures, small mouth, and micrognathia, a high, narrow palate, clenched hands with the second and fifth digits overlapping the third and fourth, small fingernails, short sternum, small pelvis with limited hip movement, and cryptorchidism in males.

Reference(s): Jones et al. [18]; Cereda and Carey [83].

2.42. Cataract

A cataract is an opacity of the crystalline lens. Cataracts can be congenital or acquired. There are many known types and genetic causes of cataracts, which can occur in a syndromic or nonsyndromic context. Prompt diagnosis can be important for optimal management.

Reference(s): Pichi et al. [84]; Messina-Baas and Cuevas-Covarrubias [85]; Stevenson et al. [44].

2.43. Noonan syndrome with multiple lentigines

Noonan syndrome with multiple lentigines (NSML), formerly sometimes called "LEOPARD syndrome" involves multiple lentigines in most patients (other skin findings can include cafe-au-lait macules), short stature, pectus deformity, distinctive facial features, and hypertrophic cardiomyopathy, as well as other features in some individuals. NSML is considered to be a RASopathy; pathogenic variants in multiple genes can cause NSML.

Reference(s): Gelb and Tartaglia [86]; Anderson [87].

2.44. Hyperbilirubinemia

Gilbert syndrome is one of a number of genetic conditions that can result in hyperbilirubinemia. Gilbert syndrome results from pathogenic variants in *UGT1A1*. Affected individuals have elevated levels of unconjugated bilirubin, which can be noticed as jaundice. The condition may manifest at birth, as well as later in life. Other genetic conditions that can cause hyperbilirubinemia (and which may be in the differential diagnosis) include Crigler-Najar, Dubin-Johnson, and Rotor syndromes.

Reference(s): Fretzayas et al. [88].

2.45. Waardenburg syndrome

Waardenburg syndrome can involve hearing loss and pigmentary changes affecting the eyes, hair, and skin. Pigmentary findings can include areas of hypopigmentation or heterochromia iridis, where the eyes are different colors. There are multiple different types of Waardenburg syndrome, and some may include other findings, such as distinctive craniofacial features, congenital anomalies affecting organs such as the GI system, heart, kidneys, and skeletal system. Pathogenic variants in multiple genes can cause Waardenburg syndrome.

Reference(s): Read and Newton [89]; Pingault et al. [90]; Jones et al. [18].

2.46. Seckel syndrome

A number of genetic conditions frequently involve overgrowth as a feature. These include syndromes such as Beckwith-Wiedemann, Marshall-Smith, Simpson-Golabi Behmel, Sotos, and Weaver, as well as others (but not Seckel syndrome). In addition to early overgrowth, these conditions typically include other syndromic features.

Reference(s): Edmondson and Kalish [91]; Brioude et al. [92]; Jones et al. [18].

2.47. Telecanthus

Telecanthus refers to wide spacing (more than 2 standard deviations for age) between the inner canthi, or the "inner corners" of the eye, where the upper and lower eyelids meet. Hypertelorism, or widely spaced eyes, refers to an increased interpupillary distance.

Reference(s): National Human Genome Research Institute: Elements of Morphology: Human Malformation Terminology [1].

2.48. Brachydactyly

Albright hereditary osteodystrophy (AHO), a disorder of GNAS inactivation, can include features such as intrauterine growth restriction, obesity, a round face, short stature, subcutaneous ossifications, and certain skeletal manifestations. These skeletal findings can include short and wide long bones in the hands and feet, and affected individuals may have brachydactyly, especially affecting the fourth and fifth digits.

Reference(s): Haldeman-Englert et al. [93]; Mantovani et al. [94].

2.49. Lipoatrophy

Congenital generalized lipodystrophy (also called Berardinelli-Seip congenital lipodystrophy) is an autosomal recessive condition that can be caused by pathogenic variants in *AGPAT2* or *BSCL2*. The condition is often diagnosed in early life. Major criteria include lipoatrophy; acromegaloid features; hepatomegaly, elevated serum triglycerides, and insulin resistance. Minor criteria include hypertrophic cardiomyopathy, intellectual disability, hirsutism, female precocious puberty, bone cysts, and phlebomegaly. There are also other known genetic lipodystrophy syndromes.

Reference(s): Hussain and Garg [95]; Van Maldegrem [96].

2.50. Nystagmus

Nystagmus refers to repetitive, involuntary eye movements. Nystagmus can be congenital or acquired. There are many possible causes of nystagmus, including albinism, cataracts, and other optic nerve or retinal disorders, as well as various neurological conditions. Nystagmus may occur in an apparently isolated or syndromic context; multiple specific genetic causes are known.

Reference(s): Gottlob [97]; Ehrt [98]; Papageorgiou et al. [99].

2.51. Rocker bottom foot

A "rocker bottom foot" (also called a congenital vertical talus) involves the presence of a prominent heel along with a convex sole contour. Rocker bottom feet may be observed in a number of different genetic conditions, including some of the more common aneuploidies, but may occur in the absence of an obvious or recognized syndrome or genetic condition.

Reference(s): National Human Genome Research Institute: Elements of Morphology: Human Malformation Terminology [1]; Jones et al. [18].

2.52. 40%

Assessment of physical findings can be a key part of the diagnostic process in someone suspected to have a genetic condition. Related to this, it is important to consider normal findings and variants that may correlate with developmental and related processes. The anterior fontanel closes by 12 months in about 38% of children and by 24 months in 96% (the median age of closure is 13.8 months). Early or late closure of the fontanels can be a clue to help inform the differential diagnosis for a patient.

Reference(s): Duc and Largo [100]; Kiesler and Ricer [101]; Stevenson et al. [44].

2.53. Tuberous sclerosis complex

Tuberous sclerosis complex (TSC) is a multisystem condition caused by heterozygous pathogenic variants (which may be inherited or de novo) in *TSC1* or *TSC2*. Clinical features of the condition can include neurologic and neuroanatomic/neoplastic manifestations, seizures, intellectual disability, renal neoplasms, cardiac rhabdomyomas and arrhythmias, pulmonary lymphangioleiomyomatosis, and a number of different dermatologic findings. These characteristic skin findings can include facial angiofibromas, hypomelanotic macules (sometimes termed "ash leaf spots"), Shagreen patches, "confetti" skin lesions, and ungual fibromas.

Reference(s): Becker and Strowd [102]; Northrup et al. [103].

2.54. Poland anomaly

Poland anomaly refers to unilateral pectoralis major absence or hypoplasia with ipsilateral anomaly of the upper limb, usually the hand. The condition is typically sporadic, but familial cases have been described. Poland anomaly can occur in an isolated or syndromic context.

Reference(s): Seyfer et al. [104]; Yiyit et al. [105]; Stevenson et al. [44].

2.55. Down syndrome

People with Down syndrome may have identifiable features on physical examination. These can include distinctive craniofacial and other features affecting different parts of the body, such as the hands and feet. A significant proportion of individuals with Down syndrome have "Brushfield spots," which are small, white, brown, or gray-appearing spots on the periphery of the iris. These are often most obvious in people with light-colored eyes.

Reference(s): Rex and Preus [106]; Berk et al. [107].

References

Chapter 2

1. National Human Genome Research Institute: Elements of Morphology: Human Malformation Terminology. https://elementsofmorphology.nih.gov/ (accessed 26 July 2021).
2. Hall, B.D., Graham, J.M. Jr., Cassidy, S.B., and Opitz, J.M. (2009). Elements of morphology: standard terminology for the periorbital region. *Am. J. Med. Genet. A* 149A: 29–39.
3. Biesecker, L.G., Aase, J.M., Clericuzio, C. et al. (2009). Elements of morphology: standard terminology for the hands and feet. *Am. J. Med. Genet. A* 149A: 93–127.
4. Mussa, A., Russo, S., Larizza, L. et al. (2016). (Epi)genotype-phenotype correlations in Beckwith-Wiedemann syndrome: a paradigm for genomic medicine. *Clin. Genet.* 89: 403–415.
5. Baroni, A. (2019). Long-wave plasma radiofrequency ablation for treatment of xanthelasma palpebrarum. *J. Cosmet. Dermatol.* 18: 121–123.
6. Rodriguez-Bujaldon, A., Vazquez-Bayo, C., Jimenez-Puya, R. et al. (2008). LEOPARD syndrome: what are cafe noir spots? *Pediatr. Dermatol.* 25: 444–448.
7. Wikimedia Commons. https://commons.wikimedia.org/wiki/File:Brushfield_eye_crop.jpg (accessed 26 July 2021).
8. Deardorff, M.A., Noon, S.E., and Krantz, I.D. (1993). Cornelia de Lange syndrome. In: *GeneReviews®* (ed. M.P. Adam, H.H. Ardinger, R.A. Pagon, et al.). Seattle, WA: University of Washington.
9. Mehta, D., Vergano, S.A., Deardorff, M. et al. (2016). Characterization of limb differences in children with Cornelia de Lange syndrome. *Am. J. Med. Genet. C Semin. Med. Genet.* 172: 155–162.
10. Jones, K.L., Jones, M.C., and del Campo, M. (2013). *Smith's Recognizable Patterns of Human Malformation*. Philadelphia, PA: Elsevier Saunders.
11. Ashwal, S., Michelson, D., Plawner, L. et al. (2009). Practice parameter: Evaluation of the child with microcephaly (an evidence-based review): report of the Quality Standards Subcommittee of the American Academy of Neurology and the Practice Committee of the Child Neurology Society. *Neurology* 73: 887–897.
12. Duerinckx, S. and Abramowicz, M. (2018). The genetics of congenitally small brains. *Semin. Cell Dev. Biol.* 76: 76–85.
13. Busche, A., Hehr, U., Sieg, P., and Gillessen-Kaesbach, G. (2016). Van der Woude and Popliteal Pterygium syndromes: broad intrafamilial variability in a three generation family with mutation in IRF6. *Am. J. Med. Genet. A* 170: 2404–2407.
14. Schutte, B.C., Saal, H.M., Goudy, S., and Leslie, E.J. (1993). IRF6-related disorders. In: *GeneReviews®* (ed. M.P. Adam, H.H. Ardinger, R.A. Pagon, et al.). Seattle, WA: University of Washington.
15. Wattendorf, D.J. and Muenke, M. (2005). Fetal alcohol spectrum disorders. *Am. Fam. Physician* 72 (279–282): 285.
16. Del Campo, M. and Jones, K.L. (2017). A review of the physical features of the fetal alcohol spectrum disorders. *Eur. J. Med. Genet.* 60: 55–64.
17. Sybert, V.P. and McCauley, E. (2004). Turner's syndrome. *N. Engl. J. Med.* 351: 1227–1238.
18. Jones, K., Jones, M., and del Campo, M. (2021). *Smith's Recognizable Patterns of Human Malformation*. Philadelphia, PA: Elsevier, Inc.

19. Stromme, P., Bjornstad, P.G., and Ramstad, K. (2002). Prevalence estimation of Williams syndrome. *J. Child Neurol.* 17: 269–271.
20. Morris, C.A., Braddock, S.R., and Council On, G. (2020). Health care supervision for children with Williams syndrome. *Pediatrics* 145: e20193761.
21. Dubourg, C., Bendavid, C., Pasquier, L. et al. (2007). Holoprosencephaly. *Orphanet J. Rare Dis.* 2: 8.
22. Solomon, B.D., Mercier, S., Velez, J.I. et al. (2010). Analysis of genotype-phenotype correlations in human holoprosencephaly. *Am. J. Med. Genet. C Semin. Med. Genet.* 154C: 133–141.
23. Agochukwu, N.B., Solomon, B.D., and Muenke, M. (2012). Impact of genetics on the diagnosis and clinical management of syndromic craniosynostoses. *Childs Nerv. Syst.* 28: 1447–1463.
24. Wenger, T.L., Hing, A.V., and Evans, K.N. (1993). Apert syndrome. In: *GeneReviews®* (ed. M.P. Adam, H.H. Ardinger, R.A. Pagon, et al.). Seattle, WA: University of Washington.
25. Pedersen, L.K., Maimburg, R.D., Hertz, J.M. et al. (2017). Moebius sequence -a multidisciplinary clinical approach. *Orphanet J. Rare Dis.* 12: 4.
26. Porter, F.D. (2008). Smith-Lemli-Opitz syndrome: pathogenesis, diagnosis and management. *Eur. J. Hum. Genet.* 16: 535–541.
27. Nowaczyk, M.J.M. and Wassif, C.A. (1993). Smith-Lemli-Opitz syndrome. In: *GeneReviews®* (ed. M.P. Adam, H.H. Ardinger, R.A. Pagon, et al.). Seattle, WA: University of Washington.
28. Lohmann, D.R. and Gallie, B.L. (1993). Retinoblastoma. In: *GeneReviews®* (ed. M.P. Adam, H.H. Ardinger, R.A. Pagon, et al.). Seattle, WA: University of Washington.
29. Summers, K.M., West, J.A., Peterson, M.M. et al. (2006). Challenges in the diagnosis of Marfan syndrome. *Med. J. Aust.* 184: 627–631.
30. Sacharow, S.J., Picker, J.D., and Levy, H.L. (1993). Homocystinuria caused by cystathionine beta-synthase deficiency. In: *GeneReviews®* (ed. M.P. Adam, H.H. Ardinger, R.A. Pagon, et al.). Seattle, WA: University of Washington.
31. Bandmann, O., Weiss, K.H., and Kaler, S.G. (2015). Wilson's disease and other neuro-logical copper disorders. *Lancet Neurol.* 14: 103–113.
32. Weiss, K.H. (1993). Wilson disease. In: *GeneReviews®* (ed. M.P. Adam, H.H. Ardinger, R.A. Pagon, et al.). Seattle, WA: University of Washington.
33. Bamshad, M., Van Heest, A.E., and Pleasure, D. (2009). Arthrogryposis: a review and update. *J. Bone Joint Surg. Am.* 91 (Suppl 4): 40–46.
34. Hall, J.G. and Kiefer, J. (2016). Arthrogryposis as a syndrome: gene ontology analysis. *Mol. Syndromol.* 7: 101–109.
35. Weksberg, R., Shuman, C., and Beckwith, J.B. (2010). Beckwith-Wiedemann syndrome. *Eur. J. Hum. Genet.* 18: 8–14.
36. Shuman, C., Beckwith, J.B., and Weksberg, R. (1993). Beckwith-Wiedemann syndrome. In: *GeneReviews®* (ed. M.P. Adam, H.H. Ardinger, R.A. Pagon, et al.). Seattle, WA: University of Washington.
37. Nussbaum, R.L., McInnes, R.R., and Willard, H.F. (2016). *Thompson & Thompson Genetics in Medicine*. Philadelphia: Elsevier.
38. Lehman, A., Wuyts, W., and Patel, M.S. (1993). Adams-Oliver syndrome. In: *GeneReviews®* (ed. M.P. Adam, H.H. Ardinger, R.A. Pagon, et al.). Seattle, WA: University of Washington.

39. Hassed, S., Li, S., Mulvihill, J. et al. (2017). Adams-Oliver syndrome review of the literature: refining the diagnostic phenotype. *Am. J. Med. Genet. A* 173: 790–800.

40. Fergelot, P., Van Belzen, M., Van Gils, J. et al. (2016). Phenotype and genotype in 52 patients with Rubinstein-Taybi syndrome caused by EP300 mutations. *Am. J. Med. Genet. A* 170: 3069–3082.

41. Stevens, C.A. (1993). Rubinstein-Taybi syndrome. In: *GeneReviews®* (ed. M.P. Adam, H.H. Ardinger, R.A. Pagon, et al.). Seattle, WA: University of Washington.

42. Evans, K.N., Sie, K.C., Hopper, R.A. et al. (2011). Robin sequence: from diagnosis to development of an effective management plan. *Pediatrics* 127: 936–948.

43. Breugem, C.C., Evans, K.N., Poets, C.F. et al. (2016). Best practices for the diagnosis and evaluation of infants with robin sequence: a clinical consensus report. *JAMA Pediatr.* 170: 894–902.

44. Stevenson, R.E., Allanson, J.G., Everman, D.B., and Solomon, B.D. (2016). *Human Malformations and Related Anomalies*. Oxford; New York: Oxford University Press).

45. Clarke, L.A. (1993). Mucopolysaccharidosis type I. In: *GeneReviews®* (ed. M.P. Adam, H.H. Ardinger, R.A. Pagon, et al.). Seattle, WA: University of Washington.

46. Pont, S.J., Robbins, J.M., Bird, T.M. et al. (2006). Congenital malformations among liveborn infants with trisomies 18 and 13. *Am. J. Med. Genet. A* 140: 1749–1756.

47. Crider, K.S., Olney, R.S., and Cragan, J.D. (2008). Trisomies 13 and 18: population prevalences, characteristics, and prenatal diagnosis, metropolitan Atlanta, 1994–2003. *Am. J. Med. Genet. A* 146A: 820–826.

48. Judge, D.P. and Dietz, H.C. (2005). Marfan's syndrome. *Lancet* 366: 1965–1976.

49. Dietz, H. (1993). Marfan syndrome. In: *GeneReviews®* (ed. M.P. Adam, H.H. Ardinger, R.A. Pagon, et al.). Seattle, WA: University of Washington.

50. Pyeritz, R.E. (2019). Marfan syndrome: improved clinical history results in expanded natural history. *Genet. Med.* 21: 1683–1690.

51. Bonnet, C., Roubertie, A., Doummar, D. et al. (2010). Developmental and benign movement disorders in childhood. *Mov. Disord.* 25: 1317–1334.

52. Meneret, A., Trouillard, O., Dunoyer, M. et al. (1993). Congenital mirror movements. In: *GeneReviews®* (ed. M.P. Adam, H.H. Ardinger, R.A. Pagon, et al.). Seattle, WA: University of Washington.

53. Ream, M. (2015). Hypomelanosis of Ito. *Handb. Clin. Neurol.* 132: 281–289.

54. McGovern, M.M., Aron, A., Brodie, S.E. et al. (2006). Natural history of type A Niemann-Pick disease: possible endpoints for therapeutic trials. *Neurology* 66: 228–232.

55. Chen, H., Chan, A.Y., Stone, D.U., and Mandal, N.A. (2014). Beyond the cherry-red spot: ocular manifestations of sphingolipid-mediated neurodegenerative and inflammatory disorders. *Surv. Ophthalmol.* 59: 64–76.

56. Toro, C., Shirvan, L., and Tifft, C. (1993). HEXA disorders. In: *GeneReviews®* (ed. M.P. Adam, H.H. Ardinger, R.A. Pagon, et al.). Seattle, WA: University of Washington.

57. Macedo, A. Jr., Rondon, A., and Ortiz, V. (2012). Hypospadias. *Curr. Opin. Urol.* 22: 447–452.

58. Eggermann, T. (2010). Russell-Silver syndrome. *Am. J. Med. Genet. C Semin. Med. Genet.* 154C: 355–364.

59. Wakeling, E.L., Brioude, F., Lokulo-Sodipe, O. et al. (2017). Diagnosis and management of Silver-Russell syndrome: first international consensus statement. *Nat. Rev. Endocrinol.* 13: 105–124.

60. Saal, H.M., Harbison, M.D., and Netchine, I. (1993). Silver-Russell syndrome. In: *GeneReviews®* (ed. M.P. Adam, H.H. Ardinger, R.A. Pagon, et al.). Seattle, WA: University of Washington.

61. Malfait, F., Francomano, C., Byers, P. et al. (2017). The 2017 international classification of the Ehlers-Danlos syndromes. *Am. J. Med. Genet. C Semin. Med. Genet.* 175: 8–26.

62. Malfait, F., Wenstrup, R., and De Paepe, A. (1993). Classic Ehlers-Danlos syndrome. In: *GeneReviews®* (ed. M.P. Adam, H.H. Ardinger, R.A. Pagon, et al.). Seattle, WA: University of Washington.

63. Hunter, A. and Soothill, P. (2002). Gastroschisis – an overview. *Prenat. Diagn.* 22: 869–873.

64. Feldkamp, M.L., Carey, J.C., and Sadler, T.W. (2007). Development of gastroschisis: review of hypotheses, a novel hypothesis, and implications for research. *Am. J. Med. Genet. A* 143A: 639–652.

65. Cooper, S.C., Flaitz, C.M., Johnston, D.A. et al. (2001). A natural history of cleidocranial dysplasia. *Am. J. Med. Genet.* 104: 1–6.

66. Dincsoy Bir, F., Dinckan, N., Guven, Y. et al. (2017). Cleidocranial dysplasia: clinical, endocrinologic and molecular findings in 15 patients from 11 families. *Eur. J. Med. Genet.* 60: 163–168.

67. Machol, K., Mendoza-Londono, R., and Lee, B. (1993). Cleidocranial dysplasia spectrum disorder. In: *GeneReviews®* (ed. M.P. Adam, H.H. Ardinger, R.A. Pagon, et al.). Seattle, WA: University of Washington.

68. Verloes, A., Drunat, S., Gressens, P., and Passemard, S. (1993). Primary autosomal recessive microcephalies and Seckel syndrome spectrum disorders – retired chapter, for historical reference only. In: *GeneReviews®* (ed. M.P. Adam, H.H. Ardinger, R.A. Pagon, et al.). Seattle, WA: University of Washington.

69. Mace, J.W., Goodman, S.I., Centerwall, W.R., and Chinnock, R.F. (1976). The child with an unusual odor. A clinical resume. *Clin. Pediatr.* 15: 57–62.

70. Rizzo, W.B. and Roth, K.S. (1994). On "being led by the nose". Rapid detection of inborn errors of metabolism. *Arch. Pediatr. Adolesc. Med.* 148: 869–872.

71. Burton, B.K. (1998). Inborn errors of metabolism in infancy: a guide to diagnosis. *Pediatrics* 102: E69.

72. Phillips, I.R. and Shephard, E.A. (1993). Primary trimethylaminuria. In: *GeneReviews®* (ed. M.P. Adam, H.H. Ardinger, R.A. Pagon, et al.). Seattle, WA: University of Washington.

73. Cerruti Mainardi, P. (2006). Cri du Chat syndrome. *Orphanet J. Rare Dis.* 1: 33.

74. Nguyen, J.M., Qualmann, K.J., Okashah, R. et al. (2015). 5p deletions: current knowledge and future directions. *Am. J. Med. Genet. C Semin. Med. Genet.* 169: 224–238.

75. Bell, D.A., Hooper, A.J., Watts, G.F., and Burnett, J.R. (2012). Mipomersen and other therapies for the treatment of severe familial hypercholesterolemia. *Vasc. Health Risk Manag.* 8: 651–659.

76. Abul-Husn, N.S., Manickam, K., Jones, L.K. et al. (2016). Genetic identification of familial hypercholesterolemia within a single U.S. health care system. *Science* 354.

77. Goyal, G., Heaney, M.L., Collin, M. et al. (2020). Erdheim-Chester disease: consensus recommendations for evaluation, diagnosis, and treatment in the molecular era. *Blood* 135: 1929–1945.

78. Kobic, A., Shah, K.K., Schmitt, A.R. et al. (2020). Erdheim-Chester disease: expanding the spectrum of cutaneous manifestations. *Br. J. Dermatol.* 182: 405–409.

79. Klimo, P. Jr., Rao, G., and Brockmeyer, D. (2007). Congenital anomalies of the cervical spine. *Neurosurg. Clin. N. Am.* 18: 463–478.

80. Colombi, M., Dordoni, C., Chiarelli, N., and Ritelli, M. (2015). Differential diagnosis and diagnostic flow chart of joint hypermobility syndrome/ehlers-danlos syndrome hypermobility type compared to other heritable connective tissue disorders. *Am. J. Med. Genet. C Semin. Med. Genet.* 169C: 6–22.

81. Verstraeten, A., Alaerts, M., Van Laer, L., and Loeys, B. (2016). Marfan syndrome and related disorders: 25 years of gene discovery. *Hum. Mutat.* 37: 524–531.

82. Meester, J.A.N., Verstraeten, A., Schepers, D. et al. (2017). Differences in manifestations of Marfan syndrome, Ehlers-Danlos syndrome, and Loeys-Dietz syndrome. *Ann. Cardiothorac. Surg.* 6: 582–594.

83. Cereda, A. and Carey, J.C. (2012). The trisomy 18 syndrome. *Orphanet J. Rare Dis.* 7: 81.

84. Pichi, F., Lembo, A., Serafino, M., and Nucci, P. (2016). Genetics of congenital cataract. *Dev. Ophthalmol.* 57: 1–14.

85. Messina-Baas, O. and Cuevas-Covarrubias, S.A. (2017). Inherited congenital cataract: a guide to suspect the genetic etiology in the cataract genesis. *Mol. Syndromol.* 8: 58–78.

86. Gelb, B.D. and Tartaglia, M. (1993). Noonan syndrome with multiple lentigines. In: *GeneReviews*® (ed. M.P. Adam, H.H. Ardinger, R.A. Pagon, et al.). Seattle, WA: University of Washington.

87. Anderson, S. (2020). Cafe au Lait Macules and associated genetic syndromes. *J. Pediatr. Health Care* 34: 71–81.

88. Fretzayas, A., Moustaki, M., Liapi, O., and Karpathios, T. (2012). Gilbert syndrome. *Eur. J. Pediatr.* 171: 11–15.

89. Read, A.P. and Newton, V.E. (1997). Waardenburg syndrome. *J. Med. Genet.* 34: 656–665.

90. Pingault, V., Ente, D., Dastot-Le Moal, F. et al. (2010). Review and update of mutations causing Waardenburg syndrome. *Hum. Mutat.* 31: 391–406.

91. Edmondson, A.C. and Kalish, J.M. (2015). Overgrowth syndromes. *J. Pediatr. Genet.* 4: 136–143.

92. Brioude, F., Toutain, A., Giabicani, E. et al. (2019). Overgrowth syndromes – clinical and molecular aspects and tumour risk. *Nat. Rev. Endocrinol.* 15: 299–311.

93. Haldeman-Englert, C.R., Hurst, A.C.E., and Levine, M.A. (1993). Disorders of GNAS inactivation. In: *GeneReviews*® (ed. M.P. Adam, H.H. Ardinger, R.A. Pagon, et al.). Seattle, WA: University of Washington.

94. Mantovani, G., Bastepe, M., Monk, D. et al. (2018). Diagnosis and management of pseudohypoparathyroidism and related disorders: first international Consensus Statement. *Nat. Rev. Endocrinol.* 14: 476–500.

95. Hussain, I. and Garg, A. (2016). Lipodystrophy syndromes. *Endocrinol. Metab. Clin. N. Am.* 45: 783–797.

96. Van Maldergem, L. (1993). Berardinelli-Seip congenital lipodystrophy. In: *GeneReviews®* (ed. M.P. Adam, H.H. Ardinger, R.A. Pagon, et al.). Seattle, WA: University of Washington.

97. Gottlob, I. (2001). Nystagmus. *Curr. Opin. Ophthalmol.* 12: 378–383.

98. Ehrt, O. (2012). Infantile and acquired nystagmus in childhood. *Eur. J. Paediatr. Neurol.* 16: 567–572.

99. Papageorgiou, E., McLean, R.J., and Gottlob, I. (2014). Nystagmus in childhood. *Pediatr. Neonatol.* 55: 341–351.

100. Duc, G. and Largo, R.H. (1986). Anterior fontanel: size and closure in term and preterm infants. *Pediatrics* 78: 904–908.

101. Kiesler, J. and Ricer, R. (2003). The abnormal fontanel. *Am. Fam. Physician* 67: 2547–2552.

102. Becker, B. and Strowd, R.E. 3rd. (2019). Phakomatoses. *Dermatol. Clin.* 37: 583–606.

103. Northrup, H., Koenig, M.K., Pearson, D.A., and Au, K.S. (1993). Tuberous sclerosis complex. In: *GeneReviews®* (ed. M.P. Adam, H.H. Ardinger, R.A. Pagon, et al.). Seattle, WA: University of Washington.

104. Seyfer, A.E., Fox, J.P., and Hamilton, C.G. (2010). Poland syndrome: evaluation and treatment of the chest wall in 63 patients. *Plast. Reconstr. Surg.* 126: 902–911.

105. Yiyit, N., Isitmangil, T., and Oksuz, S. (2015). Clinical analysis of 113 patients with Poland syndrome. *Ann. Thorac. Surg.* 99: 999–1004.

106. Rex, A.P. and Preus, M. (1982). A diagnostic index for Down syndrome. *J. Pediatr.* 100: 903–906.

107. Berk, A.T., Saatci, A.O., Ercal, M.D. et al. (1996). Ocular findings in 55 patients with Down's syndrome. *Ophthalmic Genet.* 17: 15–19.

Clinical Diagnosis and Manifestations of Specific Conditions

3

3.1. What autosomal recessive form of long QT syndrome includes sensorineural hearing loss?
   A. Alport syndrome
   B. Dravet syndrome
   C. Jervell and Lange-Nielsen syndrome
   D. Timothy syndrome

3.2. Which of the following is a typical/diagnostic feature for certain inherited cardio-genetic disorders, but NOT for familial hypercholesterolemia?
   A. Arrhythmias
   B. Early atherosclerosis
   C. High LDL cholesterol
   D. Xanthomas

3.3. Which of the following is most typical in maturity-onset diabetes of the young (MODY)?
   A. Adolescent or young adulthood onset
   B. Insulin dependence
   C. Neonatal onset
   D. Thyroid disease

3.4. Ectopia lentis occurs in approximately what percentage of people with Marfan syndrome?
   A. 1%
   B. 10%
   C. 60%
   D. 99%

3.5. Which of the following cardiac features is most frequent in individuals with Noonan syndrome?
   A. Pulmonary valve stenosis
   B. Tetralogy of Fallot
   C. Dextrocardia
   D. Dilated cardiomyopathy

3.6. An infant is born to a parent with Neurofibromatosis type 1 (NF1). In an infant with this condition, which clinical feature is most likely to be observed?
   A. Cafe-au-lait macules
   B. Dermal neurofibromas
   C. Lisch nodules
   D. Optic gliomas

3.7. A patient seen by genetics is noted to have developmental delay, obesity, postaxial polydactyly, and renal disease. What condition is most likely?
   A. Bardet-Biedl syndrome
   B. Joubert syndrome
   C. McKusick-Kaufman syndrome
   D. Senior-Loken syndrome

3.8. Current prospective data show the highest risk of what type of cancer in women with pathogenic variants in the *BRCA1* or *BRCA2* genes?
   A. Adrenal cortical
   B. Breast
   C. Ovarian
   D. Renal

Medical Genetics and Genomics: Questions for Board Review, First Edition. Benjamin D. Solomon.
© 2023 John Wiley & Sons Ltd. Published 2023 by John Wiley & Sons Ltd.

3.9. In an infant with findings consistent with VACTERL association (including radial anomalies), which of the conditions below would most likely be in the differential diagnosis?

A. Aarskog syndrome
B. Fanconi anemia
C. Prader-Willi syndrome
D. Marfan syndrome

3.10. Which condition typically includes neonatal hypotonia followed by excessive eating in childhood?

A. Angelman syndrome
B. Beckwith-Wiedemann syndrome
C. Pallister-Hall syndrome
D. Prader-Willi syndrome

3.11. Which mitochondrial condition includes pancreatic failure, sideroblastic anemia, and pancytopenia?

A. Leigh syndrome
B. Kearns-Sayre syndrome
C. Mitochondrial epilepsy with ragged red fibers (MERRF)
D. Pearson syndrome

3.12. A male with thrombocytopenia, eczema, and recurrent ear infections might be suspected of having what condition?

A. Alagille syndrome
B. Fragile X syndrome
C. Noonan syndrome
D. Wiskott-Aldrich syndrome

3.13. What is the most common condition resulting in disproportionate small stature?

A. Achondroplasia
B. Diastrophic dysplasia
C. Hypochondroplasia
D. Thanatophoric dysplasia

3.14. An infant is diagnosed with a cardiac rhabdomyoma. What condition is most likely?

A. Neurofibromatosis type 1
B. Neurofibromatosis type 2
C. Tuberous sclerosis complex
D. Zellweger syndrome

3.15. At what age does Huntington disease typically manifest?

A. 5–10 years
B. 20–30 years
C. 35–44 years
D. 55–75 years

3.16. What condition would "wormian bones" on x-ray most likely suggest?

A. Bardet-Biedl syndrome
B. Cri-du-chat syndrome
C. Osteogenesis imperfecta
D. Spinocerebellar ataxia

3.17. What syndrome is most likely in a macrosomic neonate with hypoglycemia, macroglossia, and ear pits?

A. Beckwith-Wiedemann syndrome
B. Gorlin syndrome
C. Omenn syndrome
D. Proteus syndrome

3.18. Which clinical manifestation is most likely in a man with an XYY karyotype?

A. Gonadal dysgenesis
B. Increased height
C. Infertility
D. Severe cardiac anomalies

3.19. Which can result due to hereditary pancreatitis?

A. Limb pain and parethesias
B. Low amylase or lipase
C. Increased risk of pancreatic cancer
D. Pulmonary fibrosis

3.20. Which condition would most likely manifest with early-onset cardiomyopathy?
A. Cystinosis disease
B. Gaucher disease
C. Niemann-Pick disease
D. Pompe disease

3.21. Which electrolyte anomaly (related to the condition) would be most likely in an infant with deletion 22q11.2 syndrome?
A. Hypercalcemia
B. Hyperkalemia
C. Hypocalcemia
D. Hyponatremia

3.22. A "molar tooth sign" is identified on a brain MRI. What condition would this finding suggest?
A. Ectodermal dysplasia
B. Joubert syndrome
C. Lowe syndrome
D. Townes-Brocks syndrome

3.23. What sequence can include pulmonary hypoplasia due to oligohydramnios, such as due to fetal renal anomalies?
A. Amniotic band
B. Caudal dysplasia
C. Pierre-Robin
D. Potter

3.24. Supravalvar aortic stenosis is most associated with what condition?
A. 1p36 deletion syndrome
B. Marfan syndrome
C. Miller-Dieker syndrome
D. Williams syndrome

3.25. What finding would be most likely in a patient with hereditary hemorrhagic telangiectasia?
A. Deafness
B. Developmental delay
C. Nosebleeds
D. Pancytopenia

3.26. What condition includes skin findings (e.g. facial papules), lung cysts, and renal tumors?
A. Birt-Hogg-Dubé syndrome
B. Gorlin syndrome
C. Li-Fraumeni syndrome
D. Shwachman-Diamond syndrome

3.27. What general class of conditions is due to abnormal development/destruction of the central nervous system (CNS) white matter?
A. Immunodeficiency
B. Leukodystrophy
C. Muscular dystrophy
D. Peripheral neuropathy

3.28. What syndrome involves (among other features) hypoplasia of the zygomatic bones and mandible?
A. Carpenter syndrome
B. Crouzon syndrome
C. Hydrolethalus syndrome
D. Treacher-Collins syndrome

3.29. Which of the following is observed/true in patients with prune belly syndrome?
A. Absent lower limb muscles
B. Hearing loss
C. Ophthalmologic and neuroanatomic anomalies
D. More common in males

3.30. Which X-linked condition or syndrome is more severe in females than males?
A. Aarskog syndrome
B. Craniofrontonasal dysplasia
C. Fragile X syndrome
D. Simpson-Golabi-Behmel syndrome

3.31. Which eye finding is most common in patients with CHARGE syndrome?
A. Cataract
B. Coloboma
C. Cryptophthalmos
D. Glaucoma

3.32. Fibrocystic liver disease, cystic kidney disease, polydactyly, and retinal degeneration can all be features of what class of conditions?
A. Autoinflammatory disorders
B. Ciliopathies
C. Neurocutaneous conditions
D. Progeroid conditions

3.33. Which of the following is a disorder of copper metabolism?
A. Biotinidase deficiency
B. Hypophosphatemic rickets
C. Menkes disease
D. Methylmalonic acidemia

3.34. What hepatic finding is typical of patients with Alagille syndrome?
A. Bile duct paucity
B. Hemochromatosis
C. Hepatitis A
D. Hepatoma

3.35. What cancer type is most common in people with Gorlin syndrome, a condition that can be caused by pathogenic variants in *PTCH1*?
A. Adrenocortical carcinoma
B. Basal cell carcinoma
C. Kaposi sarcoma
D. Prostate cancer

3.36. What condition would most likely be suspected in an infant with meconium ileus?
A. Cystic fibrosis
B. Maple syrup urine disease
C. Sickle cell anemia
D. Tracheoesophageal fistula

3.37. Which acronym is a term for an ophthalmologic finding associated with APC-related polyposis conditions?
A. CHRPE
B. FAP
C. MMR
D. MSI

3.38. A patient is suspected to have a genetic condition. One of the person's clinical manifestations involves "drop attacks" in which the person sometimes falls down when there is sudden stimuli. What condition might be suspected?
A. Antley-Bixler syndrome
B. Coffin-Lowry syndrome
C. Holt-Oram syndrome
D. Treacher-Collins syndrome

3.39. What condition would most likely be suspected in a child with a cleft palate, severe myopia, and hearing loss, and who has a similarly affected parent?
A. Kabuki syndrome
B. Marfan syndrome
C. Osteogenesis imperfecta
D. Stickler syndrome

3.40. Charcot-Marie-Tooth, or hereditary motor and sensory neuropathy (HMSN), primarily affects what part of the body?
A. Central nervous system
B. Liver
C. Peripheral nerves
D. Skin

3.41. What are the two most common types of congenital heart anomalies in infants with Down syndrome?
A. Aortic coarctation and Total anomalous pulmonary venous return
B. Atrial septal defect and Truncus arteriosus
C. Atrioventricular canal and Ventricular septal defect
D. Doublet outlet right ventricle and Tetralogy of Fallot

3.42. What condition is associated with the following tumors: hemangioblastoma, renal cell carcinoma, and pheochromocytoma, as well as other neoplasms?
A. Li-Fraumeni syndrome
B. Lynch syndrome
C. Tuberous sclerosis complex
D. Von Hippel-Lindau syndrome

3.43. What brain or related finding is most characteristic in patients with Miller-Dieker syndrome?
A. Anencephaly
B. Holoprosencephaly
C. Lissencephaly
D. Macrocephaly

3.44. Up to half of patients with Diamond-Blackfan anemia have what clinical feature?
A. Congenital malformations
B. Drug allergies
C. Preeclampsia
D. Seizures

3.45. What cardiac condition has ECG findings of ST segment elevation (in leads V1–V3) in the absence of structural heart disease?
A. Brugada syndrome
B. Long QT syndrome
C. Marfan syndrome
D. Short QT syndrome

3.46. What condition involves risk of bone marrow failure, malignancy, and pulmonary fibrosis, and is characterized by the triad of: dysplastic nails, lacy reticular pigmentation of the upper chest/neck, and oral leukoplakia?
A. Alpha-thalassemia
B. Dyskeratosis congenita
C. Fanconi anemia
D. Griscelli syndrome

3.47. What condition might be suspected in a patient with hematuria and hearing loss?
A. Aicardi syndrome
B. Alport syndrome
C. Long QT syndrome
D. Usher syndrome

3.48. What type of carcinoma is most associated with multiple endocrine neoplasia type 2?
A. Adrenal cortical
B. Breast
C. Medullary thyroid
D. Prostate

3.49. A child has severe developmental delay, microcephaly, and seizures. Which condition or syndrome would be most likely?
A. Alagille syndrome
B. Angelman syndrome
C. Cowden syndrome
D. Scheie syndrome

3.50. What is one of the most common causes of childhood macular degeneration?
A. Anophthalmia
B. Coloboma
C. Conjunctivitis
D. Stargardt disease

3.51. A patient with aniridia is found to have a de novo, heterozygous deletion of chromosome 11p13. Which cancer type is most associated with this condition?
A. Osteosarcoma
B. Pheochromocytoma
C. Retinoblastoma
D. Wilms tumor

3.52. Which of the following is true/typical of familial hemiplegic migraine (FMH)?
A. Caused by teratogens
B. Leads to myocardial infarction and stroke
C. Preceded by aura
D. Recessive inheritance

3.53. A term infant has severe lung disease that appears very similar to respiratory distress syndrome as would affect a very premature infant. What genetic condition is most likely?

A. Achondroplasia

B. Prader-Willi syndrome

C. Refsum disease

D. Surfactant dysfunction

3.54. A man has situs inversus, infertility, and a history of chronic airway infections. What condition is most likely?

A. Cystic fibrosis

B. Klinefelter syndrome

C. Primary ciliary dyskinesia

D. Telomere dysfunction

3.55. What condition classically involves the triad of infantile spasms, central chorioretinal lacunae, and corpus callosum agenesis?

A. Aicardi syndrome

B. Nablus syndrome

C. PHACE syndrome

D. VACTERL association

3.56. A woman has classic galactosemia, which has been very well controlled throughout life. What sequela is most likely as a result of this condition?

A. Hyperthyroidism

B. Primary ovarian insufficiency

C. Renal failure

D. Skin cancer

3.57. What term/historical name may be used to describe a variant or subtype of Lynch syndrome that includes a predisposition to certain skin tumors?

A. Gorlin syndrome

B. Mismatch repair syndrome

C. Muir-Torre syndrome

D. Turcot syndrome

3.58. What condition results from the absence of nerve cells in the muscles of the colon?

A. Hermansky-Pudlak syndrome

B. Hirschsprung disease

C. Omphalocele

D. Lynch syndrome

3.59. Which of the following conditions is best characterized as a congenital bleeding disorder?

A. Hereditary spherocytosis

B. Myelofibrosis

C. Sickle cell anemia

D. von Willebrand disease

3.60. Pierson syndrome is a rare condition that primarily affects which organs, as well as the brain?

A. Adrenals and thyroid

B. Kidneys and eyes

C. Lungs and liver

D. Skin and spleen

3.61. What finding (among other features) would be most characteristic in a patient with Fraser syndrome?

A. Acromegaly

B. Cryptophthalmos

C. Pyloric stenosis

D. Twin-twin transfusion

3.62. What condition can involve periodic pain crises, skin lesions, decreased sweating, eye cloudiness, and hearing loss, as well as other features such as stroke and kidney damage?

A. Cystinosis

B. Fabry disease

C. Gaucher disease

D. Pompe disease

3.63. A person has a pathogenic variant in the gene *NF2*. What type of neoplasm would be most associated with this finding?

A. Kaposi sarcoma

B. Optic glioma

C. Schwannoma

D. Thymoma

3.64. A young child has failure to thrive, diarrhea, vomiting, and fat malabsorption. Acanthocytosis is identified as part of the lab-based work-up. What condition is most likely?

A. Abetalipoproteinemia

B. Cystic fibrosis

C. Gaucher disease

D. Niemann-Pick disease

Chapter 3

3.65. Which of the following acronyms refers to a mitochondrially related hereditary optic neuropathy that usually manifests in young adults with bilateral, painless, subacute visual loss?

A. LHON

B. MELAS

C. MERRF

D. MNGIE

3.66. What syndrome, caused by pathogenic variants in *SALL1*, frequently involves imperforate anus, ear anomalies, and thumb malformations, as well as renal, cardiac, and other anomalies?

A. Crouzon syndrome

B. Marfan syndrome

C. Noonan syndrome

D. Townes-Brocks syndrome

3.67. An adult has a history of migraines and strokes, with later onset of dementia. Neuroimaging shows white matter lesions and subcortical infarcts. Multiple family members are also affected. What condition is most likely?

A. Alzheimer's disease

B. CADASIL

C. Frontotemporal dementia

D. Tay-Sachs

3.68. A 35 year-old male presents with back pain, hematuria, and hypertension, and is found to have multiple bilateral renal cysts. His mother underwent renal transplant. What condition would be most likely?

A. Autosomal dominant polycystic kidney disease (ADPKD)

B. Alport syndrome

C. Autosomal recessive polycystic kidney disease (ARPKD)

D. Joubert syndrome

3.69. A patient with congenital cardiac anomalies has anomalous pulmonary vein, which appears as a curved shape on chest radiograph. What is this type of anomaly called?

A. Ectopia cordis

B. Scimitar anomaly

C. Situs inversus

D. Tetralogy of Fallot

3.70. You are seeing a patient suspected to have Septo-optic dysplasia. In addition to agenesis/anomalies of the septum pellucidum and corpus callosum and optic nerve hypoplasia, what finding would you anticipate?

A. Hirschsprung disease

B. Melanoma

C. Pituitary anomalies

D. Rhizomelia

3.71. In autosomal recessive polycystic kidney disease, which of the hepatic findings listed below is most characteristic?
A. Absence of the liver
B. Fibrosis
C. Hepatitis
D. Liver cysts

3.72. A family appears to have a hereditary movement disorder involving sustained muscle contractions, which result in abnormal, repetitive movements and postures. What is the best general description for the movement disorder affecting the family?
A. Dystonia
B. Epilepsy
C. Myofibrillar myopathy
D. Paresthesias

3.73. With which condition/syndrome is pulmonary fibrosis associated?
A. Bohring-Opitz syndrome
B. Fragile X syndrome
C. Hermansky-Pudlak syndrome
D. Osteogenesis imperfecta syndrome

3.74. A two-year-old has a gait disturbance and abnormal eye movements; cerebellar atrophy is noted on MRI. Laboratory work-up shows signs of immunodeficiency. What diagnosis/syndrome is most likely?
A. Ataxia-telangiectasia
B. Bardet-Biedl syndrome
C. Severe combined immunodeficiency
D. Wiskott-Aldrich syndrome

3.75. A patient has been diagnosed with primary hyperoxaluria. What clinical feature would be most likely?
A. Autism
B. Immunodeficiency
C. Kidney stones
D. Seizures

3.76. A "lemon sign" is noted on prenatal ultrasound. What condition is most associated with this observation?
A. Gastroschisis
B. Renal agenesis
C. Spina bifida
D. Truncus arteriosus

3.77. A male child has congenital cataracts, infantile glaucoma, hypotonia, developmental delay, and renal dysfunction. What condition is most likely?
A. Cohen syndrome
B. Lowe syndrome
C. Marfan syndrome
D. Noonan syndrome

3.78. A patient had failure-to-thrive due to malabsorption, short stature, recurrent infections, and has been diagnosed with leukemia. What syndrome is most likely?
A. Diamond-Blackfan syndrome
B. Ehlers-Danlos syndrome
C. Meckel-Gruber syndrome
D. Shwachman-Diamond syndrome

3.79. A pregnant woman has a Zika virus infection. Which of the following sequelae would be most likely in the woman's child?
A. Aneuploidy
B. Cardiac anomalies
C. Microcephaly
D. Neural tube defect

3.80. An infant has anomalies on neuroimaging, including subdural hematomas, open opercula, ventriculomegaly, and white matter abnormalities. What genetic condition might be considered in the differential diagnosis?
A. Aceruloplasminemia
B. Glutaric acidemia type 1
C. Incontinentia pigmenti
D. Lowe syndrome

3.81. A child may have Fragile X syndrome. In taking a family history, what clinical feature should be specifically inquired about in the maternal grandparents?

A. Macular degeneration
B. Prematurity
C. Tremor
D. Urticaria

3.82. A patient has a genetic form of albinism. What feature, associated with decreased visual acuity, would the patient most likely have?

A. Coloboma
B. Foveal hypoplasia
C. Iris hamartomas
D. Retinitis pigmentosa

3.83. Bone marrow aspiration is done for a patient with a suspected genetic condition. The pathology report notes the presence of foam cells and sea-blue histiocytes. Which condition is most likely?

A. Dyskeratosis congenita
B. Fabry disease
C. Niemann-Pick disease
D. Refsum disease

3.84. A child with optic atrophy has been diagnosed with Wolfram syndrome. Testing for what other clinical manifestation would be warranted?

A. Diabetes mellitus
B. Hirschsprung disease
C. Hypercholesterolemia
D. Immunodeficiency

3.85. An adult patient describes progressive visual loss, which seems to be affecting her night and peripheral vision the most. Which is the most likely cause?

A. Coloboma
B. Heterochromia
C. Microphthalmia
D. Retinitis pigmentosa

Answers

3.1. C	3.18. B	3.35. B	3.52. C
3.2. A	3.19. C	3.36. A	3.53. D
3.3. A	3.20. D	3.37. A	3.54. C
3.4. C	3.21. C	3.38. B	3.55. A
3.5. A	3.22. B	3.39. D	3.56. B
3.6. A	3.23. D	3.40. C	3.57. C
3.7. A	3.24. D	3.41. C	3.58. B
3.8. B	3.25. C	3.42. D	3.59. D
3.9. B	3.26. A	3.43. C	3.60. B
3.10. D	3.27. B	3.44. A	3.61. B
3.11. D	3.28. D	3.45. A	3.62. B
3.12. D	3.29. D	3.46. B	3.63. C
3.13. A	3.30. B	3.47. B	3.64. A
3.14. C	3.31. B	3.48. C	3.65. A
3.15. C	3.32. B	3.49. B	3.66. D
3.16. C	3.33. C	3.50. D	3.67. B
3.17. A	3.34. A	3.51. D	3.68. A

3.69. B	3.74. A	3.79. C	3.84. A
3.70. C	3.75. C	3.80. B	3.85. D
3.71. B	3.76. C	3.81. C	
3.72. A	3.77. B	3.82. B	
3.73. C	3.78. D	3.83. C	

Commentary

3.1. Jervell and Lange-Nielsen syndrome

Long QT syndrome (LQTS) is a condition that involves cardiac arrhythmia (abnormal heart rhythm). Clinical manifestations can include syncope, ventricular arrhythmia, and sudden cardiac death. Depending on the type of LQTS, these manifestations may occur in infancy, childhood, or adulthood. About 75% of cases of LQTS are due to known genetic causes. Over a dozen genes have been implicated in LQTS. The inheritance for most genetic forms of LQTS is autosomal dominant, though other inheritance patterns can occur. Biallelic pathogenic variants in the genes *KCNQ1* or *KCNE1* cause Jervell and Lange-Nielsen syndrome (JLNS) – that is, the inheritance is autosomal recessive for JLNS. In addition to LQTS, patients with JLNS have congenital, bilateral, profound sensorineural hearing loss. In patients with JLNS, approximately half of cardiac events occur by age three years. The parents of affected children are almost always both heterozygous variant carriers (rare de novo variants have been reported in children) and may or may not manifest with features of LQTS.

Reference(s): Crotti et al. [1]; Tranebjærg et al. [2]; Alders and Christiaans [3].

3.2. Arrhythmias

Familial hypercholesterolemia (FH) can be caused by heterozygous pathogenic variants in a number of genes, including *APOB, LDLR*, and *PCSK9*. Biallelic (recessively inherited) pathogenic variants typically cause much more severe disease. Autosomal recessive hypercholesterolemia can also be caused by pathogenic variants in *LDLRAP1*. Common clinical features of FH include high LDL cholesterol, high total cholesterol, premature atherosclerosis, and findings on physical examination including xanthomas (areas of yellowish cholesterol buildup, which may appear on the eyelids and tendons) and corneal arcus (a white, gray, or blue lipid ring in the peripheral cornea). Identification of affected individuals is important for management, which can involve preventative measures as well as active treatment (e.g. with statins and other lipid-reducing therapies). Arrhythmias can occur in a number of other genetic conditions that affect the cardiovascular system.

Reference(s): Abul-Husn et al. [4]; Youngblom et al. [5].

3.3. Adolescent or young adulthood onset

Maturity-onset diabetes of the young (MODY) is a genetic disorder that can cause diabetes mellitus. MODY can be caused by pathogenic variants in the *HNF1A, HNF1B, HNF4A, GCK, PDX1*, and other genes. Patients can have slightly different manifestations depending on the gene involved. Pathogenic variants in certain MODY-related genes can also cause other conditions, such as neonatal diabetes mellitus. In general, it can be difficult to discern MODY from other forms of diabetes mellitus. Often, patients with MODY present in young adulthood, though can present later. Patients with MODY do not typically have autoantibodies (seen in type 1 diabetes) or traditional risk factors for diabetes such as obesity (seen in type 2 diabetes). Certain types of MODY may be ascertained due to high glucose levels on screening labs – including in pregnancy – rather than because of clinical signs and symptoms of diabetes. The inheritance for MODY is usually autosomal dominant but can also be autosomal recessive. Only a few percent (1–5%, depending on the data source) of people with diabetes mellitus have MODY, but diagnosis has important treatment implications. For example, many people with MODY will respond well to oral medications such as sulfonylureas and will not require insulin.

Reference(s): Anik et al. [6]; Hattersley and Patel [7]; Naylor et al. [8].

3.4. 60%

Marfan syndrome, which is caused by pathogenic variants in *FBN1*, can include cardiovascular, skeletal, ophthalmologic, and other manifestations. Ectopia lentis (lens dislocation) occurs in ~60% of people with Marfan syndrome. Ectopia lentis is best diagnosed via slit-lamp examination with maximal pupillary dilatation. As part of their care, people with Marfan syndrome should have annual ophthalmologic examinations. Pathogenic variants in *FBN1* can also result in other phenotypes with overlapping features of Marfan syndrome, including familial ectopia lentis, in which there is no aortic involvement.

Reference(s): Reference(s): Loeys et al. [9]; Dietz [10].

3.5. Pulmonary valve stenosis

Noonan syndrome, one of the RASopathies, often includes a distinctive craniofacial appearance, short stature and other physical examination findings, developmental delay, and several types of cardiac disease, as well as other features such as coagulopathy and other malformations. Frequent cardiac findings include pulmonary valve stenosis, hypertrophic cardiomyopathy, and atrial septal defect, though other cardiac anomalies may also occur. Pathogenic variants in one of multiple genes can cause Noonan syndrome – the most commonly implicated gene is *PTPN11*. Pathogenic variants in these and related genes can also result in conditions with overlapping clinical phenotypes.

Reference(s): Roberts et al. [11]; Allanson and Roberts [12].

3.6. Cafe-au-lait macules

Neurofibromatosis type 1 (NF1) is an autosomal dominant condition caused by pathogenic variants in the gene *NF1*. About half of affected individuals have the condition due to a de novo variant. Clinical diagnostic features involve the following (for some features, certain numbers or attributes are required): cafe-au-lait macules, neurofibromas, axillary or inguinal freckling, optic glioma, Lisch nodules, distinctive osseus lesions, and affected first-degree relatives. Many of these features are not present in infancy. Only about half of children with *NF1* without family history meet these diagnostic criteria by one year of age, though almost all meet these criteria by eight years of age.

Reference(s): Williams et al. [13]; Friedman [14].

Chapter 3

3.7. Bardet-Biedl syndrome

Bardet-Biedl syndrome (BBS), which affects multiple organ systems, is a type of ciliopathy. Characteristic features of BBS include developmental delay/intellectual disability, obesity, postaxial polydactyly, and renal disease, as well as other features, such as distinctive craniofacial features, and genitourinary (GU) anomalies. Pathogenic variants in multiple genes have been identified as causative. There are also a number of other genetic conditions that are considered ciliopathies, and many of these can have overlapping features with BBS.

Reference(s): Khan et al. [15]; Forsyth and Gunay-Aygun [16]; Jones et al. [17].

3.8. Breast

A prospective study followed thousands of women who had been found to have pathogenic variants in *BRCA1* or *BRCA2* to determine the risks for breast cancer (as well as contralateral breast cancer) and ovarian cancer. Among other findings, the study found that the cumulative risk (by age 80 years) for breast cancer was 72% for women with *BRCA1* and 69% for women with *BRCA2* pathogenic variants. The cumulative risk (by age 80 years) for ovarian cancer was 44% for women with *BRCA1* and 17% for women with *BRCA2* pathogenic variants. It is important to note that other studies, often using different methods and approaches, have found different estimates for these and other cumulative risks. Pathogenic variants in these genes also increase the risk of other cancer types.

Reference(s): Petrucelli et al. [18]; Kuchenkaecker et al. [19].

3.9. Fanconi anemia

The term "VACTERL" (or VATER) association is typically applied when a patient has at least three of the following congenital anomalies: Vertebral defects, Anal atresia, Cardiac defects, Tracheo-Esophageal fistula, Renal anomalies, and Limb abnormalities. VACTERL is an association, referring to the non-random co-occurrence of features without a recognized, unifying cause. A minority of patients with features of VACTERL (or VACTERL-H, which refers to VACTERL with Hydrocephalus) have Fanconi anemia (FA). FA can occur due to pathogenic variants in one of multiple different genes. Features of FA can include microcephaly, neurocognitive disability, short stature, abnormal skin pigmentation, and musculoskeletal anomalies (including hypoplastic thumb or radius), as well as bone marrow failure and increased risk of certain types of cancer. FA can be diagnosed through chromosome breakage studies and/or molecular testing.

Reference(s): Solomon [20]; Solomon et al. [21]; Solomon [22].

3.10. Prader-Willi syndrome

Prader-Willi syndrome (PWS) typically includes neonatal hypotonia with feeding difficulties followed by excessive eating later in childhood, developmental delay/intellectual disability and behavioral disturbances, hypogonadism, short stature, and distinctive facial features. PWS can result from multiple causes affecting chromosome 15q11.2–q13, including paternal deletion, maternal uniparental disomy (UPD), or an imprinting defect. Methylation testing of the affected region is a standard initial test when PWS is suspected in a patient.

Reference(s): Wattendorf and Muenke [23]; Driscoll et al. [24].

3.11. Pearson syndrome

Pearson syndrome is a mitochondrial DNA deletion syndrome. Features of Pearson syndrome include exocrine pancreatic dysfunction (usually manifesting as excessive stool excretion of fat), sideroblastic anemia, and pancytopenia; the condition can also include renal tubular defects. Pearson syndrome is typically fatal in infancy.

Chapter 3

Reference(s): Rötig et al. [25]; Chinnery [26].

3.12. Wiskott-Aldrich syndrome

Wiskott-Aldrich syndrome (WAS) is an X-linked recessive condition caused by pathogenic variants in the gene *WAS*. WAS typically presents in infancy; the classic clinical triad in affected males includes thrombocytopenia (manifesting as mucosal bleeding, bloody diarrhea, petechiae, and purpura), eczema, and recurrent viral and bacterial infections (especially ear infections). Later-onset manifestations can include autoimmune disease (e.g. hemolytic anemia, immune thrombocytopenic purpura, neutropenia, rheumatoid arthritis, vasculitis, and liver and kidney damage) and increased lymphoma risk.

Reference(s): Binder et al. [27]; Chandra et al. [28].

3.13. Achondroplasia

Achondroplasia is the most common condition resulting in disproportionate small stature. Clinical manifestations include relatively short arms and legs, and characteristic facial features with a large head size. Achondroplasia results from heterozygous pathogenic variants in *FGFR3*. About 80% of individuals with achondroplasia have a de novo pathogenic variant in the gene.

Reference(s): Krakow and Rimoin [29]; Legare [30].

3.14. Tuberous sclerosis complex

Tuberous sclerosis complex (TSC) is an autosomal dominant condition that can be caused by heterozygous pathogenic variants in either *TSC1* or *TSC2*. The condition can be inherited, but about two-thirds of patients have the condition due to a de novo pathogenic variant. Clinical features include skin findings (e.g. facial angiofibromas, hypomelanotic macules, Shagreen patches, and ungual fibromas), neurologic and neuroanatomic/neoplastic manifestations (including cortical dysplasia, subependymal nodules, subependymal giant cell astrocytomas, seizures, and intellectual disability), renal neoplasms and cysts, cardiac rhabdomyomas and arrhythmias, and pulmonary lymphangioleiomyomatosis.

Reference(s): Sahin et al. [31]; Northrup et al. [32].

3.15. 35–44 years

Huntington disease (HD) is an autosomal dominant progressive neurologic disorder. HD is caused by an increased number of CAG trinucleotide repeats in the gene *HTT*. The mean age of onset of is 35–44 years. Clinical features include progressive motor disability (especially chorea, but also affecting voluntary movements) and mental disturbances (cognitive decline, depression, and personality changes).

Reference(s): Walker [33]; Caron et al. [34].

3.16. Osteogenesis imperfecta

There are multiple types of Osteogenesis imperfecta (OI), as well as other conditions that share overlapping features. Clinical features can include – depending on the type of OI and the underlying cause – fractures with minimal or no trauma, short stature and bone deformity, adult-onset hearing loss, blue or gray sclerae, and dentinogenesis imperfecta. X-ray findings can include multiple fractures, "codfish vertebrae" (increased concavity of the upper and lower vertebral end plates) and osteopenia, and wormian bones. Wormian bones refer to the presence of multiple abnormal intrasutural bones.

Reference(s): Steiner et al. [35]; Jones et al. [17].

3.17. Beckwith-Wiedemann syndrome

Beckwith-Wiedemann syndrome (BWS) is a pediatric overgrowth condition that can include clinical features such as neonatal hypoglycemia, macrosomia, macroglossia, hemihyperplasia, omphalocele, visceromegaly, adrenocortical cytomegaly, renal abnormalities, and ear creases/pits. Affected patients are also at increased risk of embryonal tumors. BWS results from abnormal regulation of gene transcription affecting two imprinted domains on chromosome 11p15.5.

Reference(s): Weksberg et al. [36]; Shuman et al. [37].

3.18. Increased height

An XYY chromosome complement is relatively common, and is estimated to occur in approximately 1 in 1000 males. The occurrence is typically sporadic and incidentally diagnosed. Sequelae may include increased height and susceptibility to learning disabilities and other neurocognitive conditions such as autism and attention deficit hyperactivity disorder (ADHD). Fertility is typically preserved.

Reference(s): Leggett et al. [38]; Margari et al. [39]; Samango-Sprouse et al. [40].

3.19. Increased risk of pancreatic cancer

Pancreatitis involves inflammation of the pancreas, and can progress from acute to chronic disease. Acute pancreatitis can include attacks of abdominal pain, elevated serum amylase or lipase, and characteristic radiologic findings on abdominal imaging. Chronic pancreatitis results in irreversible pancreatic damage, and increases the risk of pancreatic cancer. Multiple genes have been identified as associated with hereditary pancreatitis; the condition may follow an autosomal dominant, autosomal recessive, or multifactorial inheritance pattern.

Reference(s): Rosendahl et al. [41]; Shelton et al. [42].

3.20. Pompe disease

Pompe disease, also known as Glycogen storage disease II, Acid maltase deficiency, or Acid α-1,4-glucosidase deficiency (there are different naming schema for the conditions based on clinical characteristics), is an autosomal recessive lysosomal storage disorder. Per one naming convention, the classic infantile form is characterized by cardiomyopathy and muscular hypotonia, while the juvenile and adult forms primarily involve skeletal muscle disease, including respiratory insufficiency. In addition to supportive care, enzyme replacement therapy has shown benefit, especially when initiated early.

Reference(s): van den Hout et al. [43]; Kishnani et al. [44]; Leslie and Bailey [45].

3.21. Hypocalcemia

Deletion 22q11.2 syndrome, sometimes called by other terms such as "DiGeorge syndrome," frequently includes congenital heart disease, palatal anomalies, distinctive facial features, learning difficulties, immune deficiency, hypocalcemia, and other findings. Hypocalcemia, related to hypoparathyroidism, is reported in up to ~80% of patients (the proportion of affected patients varies widely in the literature), and is most severe in infancy, though may be overlooked and may recur later in life. Some patients may have neonatal seizures due to hypocalcemia.

Reference(s): Cheung et al. [46]; McDonald-McGinn et al. [47]; Jones et al. [17].

3.22. Joubert syndrome

Joubert syndrome is classically and clinically defined by three main features: infantile hypotonia (which may evolve to ataxia later in childhood), developmental delay, and a distinctive brain malformation involving hypoplasia of the cerebellar vermis and brainstem, which is sometimes called the "molar tooth sign" because of its appearance on MRI. Other features in affected patients may include disordered breathing, abnormal eye movements, and anomalies affecting other organ systems such as the kidneys and eyes. Pathogenic variants in over two dozen different genes have been described as causing Joubert syndrome. Pathogenic variants in these genes can also cause allelic disorders with overlapping features.

Reference(s): Valente et al. [48]; Parisi and Glass [49]; Jones et al. [17].

3.23. Potter

A sequence is a group of related anomalies that occur due to one initial anomaly that then affects the development of other tissues or structures. Potter sequence results from oligohydramnios (low amniotic fluid), which can occur for a number of reasons, including abnormal renal development. Oligohydramnios results in findings that can include characteristic craniofacial features (sometimes called Potter facies) and pulmonary hypoplasia.

Reference(s): Jones et al. [17].

3.24. Williams syndrome

Williams syndrome results from heterozygous deletion of chromosome 7q11.23. The condition can include a distinctive appearance, neurocognitive dysfunction, endocrine disorders (including neonatal hypercalcemia, hypercalciuria, and hypothyroidism), connective tissue anomalies, and cardiovascular anomalies (including peripheral pulmonary stenosis, elastin arteriopathy, and supravalvar aortic stenosis).

Reference(s): Morris [50]; Jones et al. [17].

3.25. Nosebleeds

Hereditary hemorrhagic telangiectasia (HHT) can be due to heterozygous pathogenic variants in multiple genes, including *ACVRL1*, *ENG*, *GDF2*, and *SMAD4*; pathogenic variants in *SMAD4* have been reported in families with a combination of Juvenile polyposis syndrome and HHT. The condition results from multiple arteriovenous malformations (AVMs). Clinical manifestations include nosebleeds (epistaxis) by early adulthood, telangiectasias (found on the face, lips, tongue, chest, and fingers), and sequelae of AVMs in organs such as the lungs, liver, and brain.

Reference(s): Chung [51]; McDonald and Pyeritz [52].

3.26. Birt-Hogg-Dubé syndrome

Birt-Hogg-Dubé syndrome (BHDS) is a renal cancer syndrome due to heterozygous pathogenic variants in the gene *FLCN*. Clinical characteristics of BHDS include benign cutaneous fibrofolliculomas (skin-colored papules on the face, neck, and upper trunk) as well as other dermatologic findings, bilateral pulmonary cysts and spontaneous pneumothoraces, and kidney tumors. Renal tumors are most frequently hybrid oncocytic tumors and chromophobe renal carcinoma, but can include other tumor types, and are typically bilateral and multifocal.

Reference(s): Schmidt and Linehan [53]; Sattler and Steinlein [54].

3.27. Leukodystrophy

Leukodystrophies are a heterogeneous group of myelin disorders due to abnormal development or destruction of the white matter of the central nervous system (CNS), which may also involve the peripheral nervous system. Causes can include genetic disorders, metabolic diseases, trauma, and infection. Of the many known genetic causes, autosomal dominant, autosomal recessive (the most common inheritance pattern), and X-linked inheritance have all been described. In some types, confirmation of the molecular genetic cause of leukodystrophy may have specific management implications. Common clinical features of leukodystrophies can (depending on the underlying cause and type) include hypotonia, spasticity, motor impairment/dysfunction, MRI abnormalities, neurocognitive impairment, seizures, and effects on other organ systems such as hearing, vision, and the endocrine system.

Reference(s): Bonkowsky et al. [55]; Vanderver et al. [56].

3.28. Treacher-Collins syndrome

Treacher-Collins syndrome (TCS) (also called Mandibulofacial dysostosis or Treacher-Collins-Franceschetti syndrome) is a craniofacial condition that involves bilateral zygomatic and mandibular hypoplasia, microtia as well as frequent hearing loss, lower eyelid notching, absent lower eyelashes, and preauricular hair displacement onto the cheeks. Pathogenic variants in multiple genes can cause TCS, including *TCOF1*, *POLR1C*, and *POLR1D*.

Reference(s): Vincent et al. [57]; Katsanis and Jabs [58].

3.29. More common in males

Prune belly syndrome refers to absence or deficiency of the abdominal wall musculature, which results in the wrinkled appearance of the abdominal skin that gives the condition its name. The condition is much more common in males. In addition to the abdominal wall muscle anomalies, genitourinary anomalies are frequent, as are pulmonary anomalies, which are related to prenatal oligohydramnios. The cause(s) are incompletely understood, though some Mendelian forms have been identified.

Reference(s): Hassett et al. [59]; Stevenson et al. [60].

3.30. Craniofrontonasal dysplasia

Craniofrontonasal dysplasia is an X-linked condition due to pathogenic variants in *EFNB1*. Females are more severely affected than males. In females, the condition often includes coronal craniosynostosis, hypertelorism, clefting of the nasal tip, and additional skeletal and other anomalies. Males are typically more mildly affected and may only have hypertelorism. *EFNB1* encodes a protein whose roles involve cell surface properties and cellular interactions. The reason that females are more severely affected is thought to have to do with a process known as cellular interference. According to this explanation, random X inactivation in affected females leads to "functional mosaicism" between populations of cells with and without the variant. The interactions between these different cell populations lead to the more severe condition in females. This observation has been supported by the observation that mosaic males are more severely affected than non-mosaic males.

Reference(s): Twigg et al. [61]; Twigg et al. [62].

3.31. Coloboma

CHARGE syndrome is caused by heterozygous pathogenic variants in the gene *CHD7*. The term CHARGE is an acronym describing the main clinical features of the condition: Coloboma, Heart Defects, choanal Atresia, Retarded growth and development, Genital abnormalities, and Ear anomalies. Colobomas, which are found in up to 90% of patients, can be unilateral or bilateral, and can affect the iris, retina-choroid, and disc, and may be accompanied by microphthalmia.

Reference(s): Bergman et al. [63]; Ravenswaaij-Arts et al. [64]; Jones et al. [17].

3.32. Ciliopathies

The broad class of conditions known as "ciliopathies" refers to conditions that involve dysfunction of the cilium, a hairlike organelle. Ciliopathies include conditions like BBS, Jeune syndrome, Joubert syndrome, McKusick-Kaufman syndrome, and Meckel-Gruber syndrome. Hundreds of genes are known to be involved in ciliopathies. Relatively common systemic manifestations can include, depending on the exact gene and condition, several types of renal disease (including polycystic kidney disease, nephronophthisis, and renal dysplasia), polydactyly, congenital fibrocystic diseases of the liver, and retinal degeneration.

Reference(s): Hildebrandt et al. [65]; Reiter and Leroux [66].

3.33. Menkes disease

Menkes disease is an X-linked disorder caused by pathogenic variants in the gene *ATP7A*, which encodes a copper-transporting ATPase. Classic Menkes disease is observed in male infants who appear healthy until about 2–3 months of age, and then demonstrate failure to thrive with loss of developmental milestones, hypotonia, and seizures, along with hair changes including short, sparse, twisted, and lightly pigmented hair. In addition to molecular genetic findings, patients have low serum copper and ceruloplasmin concentrations. *ATP7A* variants also cause Occipital horn syndrome and Distal motor neuropathy.

Reference(s): Kaler [67]; Ferreira and Gahl [68]; Jones et al. [17].

3.34. Bile duct paucity

Alagille syndrome is an autosomal dominant condition due to heterozygous pathogenic variants affecting the genes *JAG1* and *NOTCH2*. Clinical criteria for Alagille syndrome include cholestasis due to bile duct paucity, which can be identified on liver biopsy, and which is found in about 90% of individuals, though not in infancy. Other major features include cardiac defects (especially stenosis of the peripheral pulmonary artery and its branches), skeletal abnormalities (especially butterfly vertebrae), ophthalmologic abnormalities (especially posterior embryotoxon), and characteristic facial features. Other anomalies, such as renal and vascular defects, are also described.

Reference(s): Saleh et al. [69]; Spinner et al. [70].

3.35. Basal cell carcinoma

Nevoid basal cell carcinoma syndrome (NBCCS), which may also be called Gorlin syndrome, Gorlin-Goltz syndrome, or Basal cell nevus syndrome, includes multiple basal cell carcinomas as well as additional findings affecting the neurologic, ophthalmologic, skeletal, and other systems, including jaw keratocysts and palmar/plantar pits. Basal cell carcinomas arise at a median age of 20 years, and patients are at risk of other neoplasms, including medulloblastoma and ovarian and cardiac fibromas. Heterozygous pathogenic variants in the gene *PTCH1* cause NBCCS/Gorlin syndrome. A smaller number of cases have been reported with pathogenic variants in *SUFU*, and *PTCH2* has been suggested to be involved as well in rare cases.

Reference(s): Evans and Farndon [71].

3.36. Cystic fibrosis

Cystic fibrosis (CF) is an autosomal recessive condition due to pathogenic variants in the *CFTR* gene, which encodes the cystic fibrosis transmembrane conductance regulator protein. CF results in multi-organ sequelae due to effects on the epithelia of the exocrine pancreas, exocrine sweat glands, hepatobiliary system, intestine, male genital tract, and respiratory tract. Meconium ileus, which refers to bowel obstruction caused by thicker/stickier meconium, occurs in ~15–20% of newborns with CF. The diagnosis of CF can be made by identifying a combination of clinical and laboratory-based features.

Reference(s): Carlyle et al. [72]; Ong et al. [73].

3.37. CHRPE

APC-related polyposis conditions are due, as the name implies, to heterozygous pathogenic variants (mutations) in the *APC* gene. These conditions include Familial adenomatous polyposis (FAP), attenuated FAP, and Gastric adenocarcinoma and proximal polyposis of the stomach (GAPPS). FAP involves thousands of adenomatous colonic polyps and risk of colon cancer; polyps can also affect the gastric fundus and duodenum. Other features can include dental anomalies, desmoid tumors, osteomas, and an ophthalmologic finding called congenital hypertrophy of the retinal pigment epithelium (CHRPE). CHRPE has been described in ~75% of patients with FAP, and refers to asymptomatic flat, pigmented retinal lesions.

Reference(s): Half et al. [74]; Jasperson et al. [75].

3.38. Coffin-Lowry syndrome

Coffin-Lowry syndrome (CLS) is an X-linked condition that includes intellectual disability, distinctive facial and other features (e.g. tapering digits), skeletal, and cardiac anomalies. About 20% of patients have stimulus-induced drop attacks, which involves collapse – without loss of consciousness – due to stimuli. CLS is caused by pathogenic variants in *RPS6KA3*.

Reference(s): Rogers and Abidi [76].

3.39. Stickler syndrome

Stickler syndrome is a connective tissue disorder. Common clinical include midface underdevelopment and cleft palate, ophthalmologic findings (including myopia, cataract, and retinal detachment), conductive and sensorineural hearing loss, and spondyloepiphyseal dysplasia and early arthritis. Stickler syndrome can be inherited in an autosomal or autosomal recessive manner. Some general genotype–phenotype correlations based on the underlying gene involved have been described.

Reference(s): Robin et al. [77]; Jones et al. [17].

3.40. Peripheral nerves

Charcot-Marie-Tooth (CMT), also known as Hereditary motor and sensory neuropathy (HMSN), is a relatively common inherited neurologic condition. CMT affects the peripheral nerves (both motor and sensory), and can affect activities such as walking, speaking, breathing, and swallowing. The severity of clinical manifestations, which usually occur in adolescence or early adulthood and progress gradually, can be highly variable. Many different genes are known to be involved in CMT, and autosomal dominant, autosomal recessive, and X-linked inheritance have been described. CMT-related genes encode proteins that are involved in the structure and function of the peripheral nerve axon or myelin sheath.

Reference(s): Bird [78].

3.41. Atrioventricular canal and Ventricular septal defect

About half of infants with Down syndrome (DS) have congenital heart anomalies. According to most studies, the two most common types are atrioventricular (AV) canals (also known as atrioventricular septal defects or endocardial cushion defects) and ventricular septal defects (VSDs), though atrial septal defects (ASDs) as well as other heart anomalies are also relatively common compared to infants without DS. The reported prevalences of the various congenital heart anomalies vary among different studies and populations and over time, which may be related to a variety of factors.

Reference(s): Bergström et al. [79]; Diogenes et al. [80].

3.42. Von-Hippel Lindau

Von-Hippel Lindau is an autosomal dominant condition caused by pathogenic variants in the *VHL* tumor suppressor gene. Affected individuals may have multiple neoplasms, including brain, retinal, and spinal hemangioblastoma, clear cell renal cell carcinoma, pheochromocytoma, neuroendocrine tumors, and endolymphatic sac tumors, as well as broad ligament, epididymal, pancreatic, and cysts. While most cases are inherited, about 20% of patients have de novo pathogenic variants. Due to the high risk of neoplasms and related sequelae, surveillance for these manifestations starting in early childhood has been recommended.

Reference(s): Maher et al. [81]; van Leeuwaarde et al. [82].

3.43. Lissencephaly

Miller-Dieker syndrome is a condition caused by heterozygous deletion of 17p13.3. The condition often includes a distinctive facial appearance, lissencephaly, seizures, and neurocognitive impairment. Patients may also have other features. Lissencephaly is attributed to loss of the *LIS1* gene, which is on the affected region of chromosome 17p13.3. Separate from Miller-Dieker syndrome, people with pathogenic variants affecting only *LIS1* may have lissencephaly.

Reference(s): Dobyns et al. [83]; Jones et al. [17].

3.44. Congenital malformations

Diamond-Blackfan anemia (DBA) involves severe anemia, congenital malformations (in up to about 50% of patients), and growth retardation (in about 30% of patients). Congenital malformations often involve the craniofacies, limbs, cardiac, and genitourinary systems. DBA can also involve other manifestations such as increased risk for certain types of cancer. DBA can be inherited in an autosomal dominant or X-linked manner, and de novo variants are relatively frequent causes of disease. Multiple genes have been shown to be involved.

Reference(s): Da Costa et al. [84]; Sieff [85].

3.45. Brugada syndrome

Brugada syndrome is an arrhythmia syndrome that involves risk of sudden death. Findings include ST segment elevation in leads V1–V3 on ECG in the absence of structural heart disease. The condition usually, but not always, presents in adulthood. Many genes have been implicated, but the evidence appears mixed for some genes, and reassessing this evidence is an area of investigation.

Reference(s): Brugada et al. [86]; Hosseini et al. [87].

3.46. Dyskeratosis congenita

Dyskeratosis congenita (DC) is a disorder of telomere biology. DC has a broad phenotypic spectrum and may be recognized by the triad of dysplastic nails, lacy reticular pigmentation of the upper chest/neck, and oral leukoplakia, though this "classic" triad may not be present in all individuals. The condition includes increased risk for bone marrow failure, myelodysplastic syndrome and hematologic malignancies, solid tumors, and pulmonary fibrosis. Pathogenic variants in multiple genes have been identified as causative.

Reference(s): Fernández Garcia et al. [88]; Savage [89].

3.47. Alport syndrome

Alport syndrome involves renal, hearing, and eye anomalies. Manifestations typically include progressive renal insufficiency, progressive sensorineural hearing loss, and variable ocular anomalies that may involve the almost pathognomonic finding of anterior lenticonus. Pathogenic variants in *COL4A3*, *COL4A4*, or *COL4A5* can cause Alport syndrome. Depending on the underlying gene, the inheritance can be X-linked (the most common inheritance pattern), autosomal dominant, or autosomal recessive.

Reference(s): Kashtan [90]; Kashtan [91].

3.48. Medullary thyroid

Multiple endocrine neoplasia (MEN) refers to a group of conditions that can cause endocrine cancer. There are multiple types and subtypes. In MEN type 2, the most common type of cancer is medullary thyroid carcinoma (MTC). MEN type 2 is divided into types 2A, 2B, and Familial medullary thyroid carcinoma (FMTC). MEN 2A can involve MTC, pheochromocytoma, and hyperparathyroidism. MEN 2B can include MTC as well as findings such as a distinctive facial appearance, mucosal neuromas of the lips and tongue, intestinal ganglioneuromas, and a Marfanoid habitus. FMTC involves a predisposition to MTC. MEN 2 is caused by heterozygous pathogenic variants in the *RET* gene.

Reference(s): Eng [92].

3.49. Angelman syndrome

Angelman syndrome typically involves severe developmental delay (manifesting at around 6 months of age), speech impairment, movement/balance disorder, specific behavioral characteristics (e.g. frequent laughing/smiling, excitability, and hand-flapping), microcephaly, and seizures, among other features. Angelman syndrome occurs due to abnormal or deficient UBE3A expression or function, which can be caused by several different types of genetic/epigenetic changes.

Reference(s): Dagli et al. [93]; Jones et al. [17].

3.50. Stargardt disease

Stargardt disease is an inherited retinal disorder, and the most common inherited macular dystrophy. The condition results from loss of photoreceptor cells in the macula (the central portion of the retina). In affected patients, visual loss typically manifests in childhood or adolescence, though may be later. One hallmark of the condition is loss of central vision. The most common cause of Stargardt disease is pathogenic variants in the gene ABCA4.

Reference(s): Altschwager et al. [94]; Tanna et al. [95].

3.51. Wilms tumor

Heterozygous deletions affecting chromosome 11p13 including the *PAX6* and *WT1* genes can cause a condition called "WAGR syndrome." In addition to aniridia (related to loss of *PAX6*) and increased risk of Wilms tumor (related to loss of *WT1*), the condition can involve GU anomalies and intellectual disability.

Reference(s): Fischbach et al. [96]; Moosajee et al. [97].

3.52. Preceded by aura

Hemiplegic migraine (HM) is a type of migraine. HM includes aura, which can include visual changes (such as blind spots, double vision, and flashing lights or lines), numbness or weakness on one side of the body, and speech changes, fatigue, and other symptoms. HM is called Familial HM (FHM) when other relatives are affected and Sporadic HM (SHM) if not. Based on family history, about half of people with HM have FHM. FHM is inherited in an autosomal dominant manner; multiple genes are known to be involved. Accurate diagnosis is important for management, as treatment for FHM may be different than for other migraine types.

Reference(s): Russell and Ducros [98]; Jen [99].

3.53. Surfactant dysfunction

Surfactant dysfunction is a genetic condition in which affected infants have severe, diffuse lung disease that clinically and radiographically resembles respiratory distress syndrome affecting premature infants. Pathogenic variants in several genes have been identified as causing the condition. Pathogenic variants in some of the involved genes can result in later-onset pulmonary disease as well as neonatal surfactant dysfunction.

Reference(s): Gower and Nogee [100]; Turcu et al. [101].

3.54. Primary ciliary dyskinesia

Primary ciliary dyskinesia (PCD) can involve situs abnormalities, infertility due to abnormal sperm motility, and chronic respiratory disease. PCD with "situs inversus totalis" is sometimes referred to as Kartagener syndrome. Pathogenic variants in dozens of different genes can result in PCD. Diagnosis can be very important for optimal medical management. For example, special care may be required for optimal respiratory health.

Reference(s): Lucas et al. [102]; Mirra et al. [103]; Zariwala et al. [104].

3.55. Aicardi syndrome

Aicardi syndrome is classically characterized by the triad of infantile spasms, central chorioretinal lacunae, and agenesis of the corpus callosum; other features are also described. The condition only affects females, though 47,XXY males with Aicardi syndrome have been described. The cause(s) of Aicardi syndrome are poorly understood.

Reference(s): Wong and Sutton [105]; Sutton and Van den Veyver [106].

3.56. Primary ovarian insufficiency

Classic galactosemia is caused by deficiency of the enzyme galactose-1-phosphate uridylyltransferase, which is due to biallelic pathogenic variants in *GALT*. Galactosemia may also be caused by variants in other genes. The most common long-term complication in women with classic galactosemia is primary or premature ovarian insufficiency (POI). Over 80% of women with classic galactosemia are affected by POI even when the condition is diagnosed neonatally and the patients follow careful lifelong dietary galactose restriction.

Reference(s): Fridovich-Keil et al. [107]; Berry [108].

3.57. Muir-Torre syndrome

"Muir-Torre syndrome" is a historical term that may be used to describe a variant or subtype of Lynch syndrome that involves the presence of sebaceous skin neoplasms. These neoplasms can include sebaceous adenomas, sebaceous epitheliomas, sebaceous carcinomas, and keratoacanthomas. The condition, which is usually inherited in an autosomal dominant fashion, can be due to pathogenic variants in mismatch repair genes. In one study, Muir-Torre syndrome was observed in about 9% of a cohort of patients with Lynch syndrome.

Reference(s): Misago and Narisawa [109]; South et al. [110]; Idos and Valle [111].

3.58. Hirschsprung disease

Hirschsprung disease (also referred to as congenital intestinal aganglionosis) occurs in about 1 in 500 births. The condition involves the absence of neuronal ganglion cells from the colonic muscles. Hirschsprung disease can result from cytogenomic anomalies, can occur in the context of a genetic syndrome with manifestations affecting multiple organ systems, or result from pathogenic variants in a number of known genes that can cause isolated (nonsyndromic) Hirschsprung disease. Currently, many cases are of unknown etiology.

Reference(s): Parisi [112]; Stevenson et al. [60].

3.59. von Willebrand disease

von Willebrand disease is a congenital bleeding disorder. The condition is caused by pathogenic variants affecting the *VWF* gene, which results in defective or deficient levels of von Willebrand factor in the plasma. There are several types and subtypes of the condition.

Reference(s): Leebeek and Eikenboom [113]; Swami and Kaur [114].

3.60. Kidneys and eyes

Pierson syndrome (not to be confused with Pearson syndrome, a mitochondrial disease involving sideroblastic anemia and exocrine pancreas dysfunction) is a rare autosomal recessive disorder caused by pathogenic variants in *LAMB2*. The condition, which is usually severe, affects the kidneys and the eyes (as well as the brain).

Specifically, renal manifestations can include congenital nephrotic syndrome with diffuse mesangial sclerosis; eye anomalies can include microcoria and hypoplasia of the ciliary and pupillary muscles.

Reference(s): Zenker et al. [115]; Matejas et al. [116].

3.61. Cryptophthalmos

Fraser syndrome is a multi-malformation condition that can be caused by pathogenic variants in multiple genes, including *FRAS1*, *FREM2*, and *GRIP1*. Characteristic features can include cryptophthalmos, cutaneous syndactyly, and genitourinary anomalies, as well as other features, such as ear and other craniofacial anomalies. Cryptophthalmos refers to an ocular anomaly in which the eyes are completely covered with skin, and can also be malformed.

Reference(s): Jadeja et al. [117]; Tessier et al. [118]; Jones et al. [17].

3.62. Fabry disease

Fabry disease is an X-linked lysosomal storage disease caused by pathogenic variants in *GLA*. Classic, atypical, and late-onset forms have been described. Manifestations can affect many organ systems, and can include periodic pain crises affecting the extremities, vascular skin lesions, decreased sweating, opacities of the cornea or lens, hearing loss, stroke, left ventricular hypertrophy, and renal insufficiency. Diagnosis is important to be able to appropriately manage the condition, including to prevent complications such as through enzyme replacement therapy.

Reference(s): Ferreira and Gahl [119]; Mehta and Hughes [120]; Wanner et al. [121].

3.63. Schwannoma

Neurofibromatosis 2 (NF2), which is caused by heterozygous pathogenic variants in *NF2*, frequently involves vestibular schwannomas. These neoplasms are present in almost all affected individuals by 30 years of age. Schwannomas affecting other nerves, as well as other neoplasms and manifestations, may also occur in affected individuals.

Reference(s): Baser et al. [122]; Evans [123].

3.64. Abetalipoproteinemia

Abetalipoproteinemia (also called Bassen-Kornzweig syndrome) is an autosomal recessive disorder caused by pathogenic variants in *MTTP*. The condition often manifests in infancy with failure to thrive, diarrhea, vomiting, and fat malabsorption. Work-up may reveal acanthocytosis, or irregularly spiculated erythrocytes visible on peripheral blood smear. If untreated, the condition can lead to sequelae affecting multiple organ systems, including visual loss, neurologic and muscular effects, and coagulopathy. Management includes dietary modifications (e.g. low-fat diet supplemented with essential fatty acids and fat-soluble vitamins).

Reference(s): Zamel et al. [124]; Jung et al. [125]; Lee and Hegele [126]; Burnett et al. [127].

3.65. LHON

Leber hereditary optic neuropathy (LHON) typically manifests in young adults as bilateral, painless, subacute visual loss. Individuals may also have other findings, including neurologic, muscular, and cardiac sequelae. The condition is more common in males; the most frequently identified cause involves specific mitochondrial variants.

Reference(s): Yu-Wai-Man et al. [128].

3.66. Townes-Brocks syndrome

Townes-Brocks syndrome is caused by heterozygous pathogenic variants in *SALL1*. The condition frequently involves imperforate anus, ear anomalies (including physical anomalies as well as hearing loss), and malformations of the thumbs. Renal and cardiac anomalies are also common, and patients may have anomalies affecting other organ systems, such as the eye.

Reference(s): Kohlhase et al. [129]; Bozal-Basterra et al. [130].

3.67. CADASIL

CADASIL is an acronym that stands for Cerebral Autosomal Dominant Arteriopathy with Subcortical Infarcts and Leukoencephalopathy. The condition usually manifests in mid-adulthood with ischemic strokes and cognitive decline, migraine, and other neuropsychiatric sequelae. Neuroimaging typically shows diffuse lesions affecting the white matter and subcortical infarcts. CADASIL is caused by heterozygous pathogenic variants in *NOTCH3*.

Reference(s): Wang [131]; Hack et al. [132].

3.68. Autosomal dominant polycystic kidney disease (ADPKD)

Autosomal dominant polycystic kidney disease (ADPKD) can present at different ages in adulthood (but can also manifest much earlier). The condition primarily involves bilateral renal cysts, liver cysts, and risk of intracranial aneurysms, though patients may have other manifestations as well. Patients may be identified because of known family history, but may also present with kidney pain, hematuria, and hypertension, as well as other renal sequelae such as urinary tract infections and kidney stones. ADPKD can be caused by pathogenic variants in several known genes.

Reference(s): Harris et al. [133]; Bergmann et al. [134].

3.69. Scimitar anomaly

A scimitar anomaly refers to a certain type of anomalous pulmonary vein, with the name deriving from the appearance of the anomalous vein on chest radiograph. Scimitar anomaly is typically associated with other cardiovascular and pulmonary anomalies. Depending on the severity, the overall presentation can range from severe neonatal manifestations to an incidental finding in adulthood.

Reference(s): Stevenson et al. [60].

3.70. Pituitary anomalies

Septo-optic dysplasia (SOD) includes the triad of agenesis/anomalies of the septum pellucidum and corpus callosum, optic nerve hypoplasia, and pituitary/hypothalamic anomalies. Other clinical features may be present as well. Pathogenic variants in multiple genes have been reported as causative.

Reference(s): Fard et al. [135]; Sataite et al. [136].

3.71. Fibrosis

Autosomal recessive polycystic kidney disease (ARPKD) may present in the neonatal period with enlarged echogenic kidneys; patients frequently have pulmonary hypoplasia due to oligohydramnios. While histologic evidence of liver fibrosis is reported to be invariably present about birth, about half of infants have clinical evidence of liver involvement at the time of diagnosis. ARPKD can be caused by biallelic pathogenic variants in the *PKHD1* gene.

Reference(s): Bergmann et al. [134]; Sweeney and Avner [137].

3.72. Dystonia

The term dystonia refers to a movement disorder involving muscle contractions, which can be sustained or intermittent, which result in abnormal, often repetitive movements or postures, and which may be associated with tremor. There are many types of dystonia, and many different genetic and nongenetic causes. The onset of hereditary forms of dystonia can range from neonatal to adult-onset presentations, and the severity and course of these conditions can vary considerably.

Reference(s): Klein et al. [138]; Newby et al. [139]; Meijer and Pearson [140].

3.73. Hermansky-Pudlak syndrome

Hermansky-Pudlak syndrome (HPS) is an autosomal recessive condition that can be caused by pathogenic variants in multiple genes. The condition may include oculocutaneous albinism (OCA), bleeding diathesis, and additional features such as granulomatous colitis, immunodeficiency, and pulmonary fibrosis. In individuals with HPS, pulmonary fibrosis can be similar to idiopathic pulmonary fibrosis, but manifests at a younger age.

Reference(s): El-Chemaly and Young [141]; Vicary et al. [142]; Huizing et al. [143].

3.74. Ataxia-telangiectasia

Ataxia-telangiectasia (A-T) is an autosomal recessive disorder caused by biallelic pathogenic variants in the *ATM*. A-T can include clinical and radiologic signs of cerebellar degeneration (the onset is typically from one to four years of age), conjunctival telangiectasia, immunodeficiency, increased risk of cancer (especially hematologic cancer), and radiation sensitivity.

Reference(s): Gatti and Perlman [144]; Rothblum-Oviatt et al. [145].

3.75. Kidney stones

Primary hyperoxaluria is a type of inborn error of metabolism that leads to high levels of urine and serum oxalate. This results in the deposition of calcium oxalate crystals in multiple organs, including as kidney stones. There are multiple types of primary hyperoxaluria; pathogenic variants in several different genes can be causative. Diagnosis is important for optimal management, including to help ameliorate long-term renal damage.

Reference(s): Cochat and Rumsby [146]; Ben-Shalom and Frishberg [147].

3.76. Spina bifida

The "lemon sign" refers to the observation of indentation affecting the frontal bone of the skull, which results in a lemon-shaped skull shape. Multiple clinical conditions can correlate with the presence of the lemon sign; this sign is observed in most fetuses affected by spina bifida.

Reference(s): Nyberg et al. [148]; Van den Hof et al. [149]; Thomas [150].

3.77. Lowe syndrome

Lowe syndrome (also called Oculocerebrorenal syndrome) is an X-linked condition caused by pathogenic variants in *OCRL*. Affected males frequently have congenital cataracts, infantile glaucoma, hypotonia, intellectual disability, and renal disease. Most females with a causative pathogenic variant develop characteristic eye findings.

Reference(s): Bökenkamp and Ludwig [151]; Lewis et al. [152].

3.78. Shwachman-Diamond syndrome

Shwachman-Diamond syndrome is an inherited bone marrow failure syndrome characterized by exocrine pancreatic dysfunction (which can lead to malabsorption and failure-to-thrive), neutropenia with predisposition to bone marrow failure, risk of myelodsyplastic syndrome and leukemia, short stature, and frequent infections. The condition can be caused by pathogenic variants in several identified genes; the most commonly involved gene is *SBDS*.

Reference(s): Nelson and Myers [153]; Nelson and Myers [154].

3.79. Microcephaly

Congenital Zika syndrome can result in a range of fetal sequelae, including microcephaly, which is due to fetal brain disruption sequence. Other findings (some of which are related to microcephaly) can include brain abnormalities, ocular abnormalities, intrauterine growth restriction, and congenital contractures; affected individuals may be affected by seizures and neurodevelopmental anomalies. Studies have provided varying estimates of risks to the fetus, but the risk appears highest in the first trimester of pregnancy.

Reference(s): Krow-Lucal et al. [155]; Poma et al. [156]; Musso et al. [157].

3.80. Glutaric acidemia type 1

Glutaric acidemia type 1, which is also known as Glutaric aciduria type 1, is an autosomal recessive inborn error of metabolism. The natural history can involve macrocephaly, encephalopathic crises, and chronic neurologic disease. Findings on neuroimaging can include open opercula, widened CSF spaces/ventriculomegaly, attenuated basal ganglia signal, white matter abnormalities, and subdural hemorrhage, though the latter finding appears to be less common than the others listed, and almost always occurs along with other neuroimaging anomalies. Timely diagnosis is important in order to implement appropriate dietary and metabolic treatment, including related to emergency care.

Reference(s): Vester et al. [158]; Vester et al. [159]; Larson and Goodman [160].

3.81. Tremor

Fragile X syndrome (FXS), the most common form of inherited intellectual disability, is an X-linked disorder caused by an increased number of CGG trinucleotide repeats in the *FMR1* gene. Based on the number of trinucleotide repeats present, alleles may be classified as normal, intermediate, premutation, or full mutation. A premutation allele may expand to a full mutation allele when passed down from a mother to a child. In addition, premutation alleles can cause Fragile X tremor ataxia syndrome (FXTAS), which involves late-onset cerebellar ataxia and tremor, or FMR1-related primary ovarian insufficiency.

Reference(s): Bagni et al. [161]; Hunter et al. [162].

3.82. Foveal hypoplasia

There are multiple different genetic forms/causes of albinism, which can occur in syndromic or nonsyndromic contexts. In general, OCA involves absent or decreased melanin pigment. This affects the pigmentation of the skin, hair, and eyes. The fovea refers to a small retinal "depression," and is the part of the eye with the highest visual acuity. Foveal hypoplasia, which occurs in albinism and is associated with decreased visual acuity, refers to a lack of development of the fovea.

Reference(s): Lewis [163]; Kondo [164].

3.83. Niemann-Pick disease

Niemann-Pick disease (NPD) includes several conditions that can involve clinical features such as CNS involvement, hepatosplenomegaly, and pulmonary insufficiency. Among these conditions, which can have different clinical presentations, NPD types A and B involve deficiency of the enzyme acid sphingomyelinase, while type C is due to defective cholesterol transport. Among other signs, laboratory-based features of NPD can include "foam cells" (lipid-laden macrophages) and sea-blue histiocytes observed on pathological examination of bone marrow aspirate.

Reference(s): Brady et al. [165]; Schuchman and Desnick [166].

3.84. Diabetes mellitus

Wolfram syndrome is an autosomal recessive condition caused by pathogenic variants in *WFS1*. The condition can involve multiple manifestations, including optic atrophy, hearing loss, diabetes mellitus and other endocrine abnormalities, and neurodegeneration, as well as other findings.

Reference(s): Tranebjærg et al. [167].

3.85. Retinitis pigmentosa

Retinitis pigmentosa (RP) is an ophthalmologic condition that involves abnormalities of the retinal rods and cones (photoreceptors), causing progressive visual loss. RP can occur in a nonsyndromic or syndromic context. RP has a great deal of locus (genetic) heterogeneity – that is, pathogenic variants in over 50 reported genes can cause the disease. Recessive, dominant, and X-linked inheritance have been described, and RP can also occur in the context of certain mitochondrial conditions. Common clinical manifestations of RP include night blindness and loss of peripheral vision.

Reference(s): Fahim et al. [168].

References

1. Crotti, L., Celano, G., Dagradi, F., and Schwartz, P.J. (2008). Congenital long QT syndrome. *Orphanet J. Rare Dis.* 3: 18.
2. Tranebjaerg, L., Samson, R.A., and Green, G.E. (1993). Jervell and Lange-Nielsen syndrome. In: *GeneReviews®* (ed. M.P. Adam, H.H. Ardinger, R.A. Pagon, et al.). Seattle, WA: University of Washington.
3. Alders, M., Bikker, H., and Christiaans, I. (1993). Long QT syndrome. In: *GeneReviews®* (ed. M.P. Adam, H.H. Ardinger, R.A. Pagon, et al.). Seattle, WA: University of Washington.
4. Abul-Husn, N.S., Manickam, K., Jones, L.K. et al. (2016). Genetic identification of familial hypercholesterolemia within a single U.S. health care system. *Science* 354: 1550.

5. Youngblom, E., Pariani, M., and Knowles, J.W. (1993). Familial hypercholesterolemia. In: *GeneReviews*® (ed. M.P. Adam, H.H. Ardinger, R.A. Pagon, et al.). Seattle, WA: University of Washington.

6. Anik, A., Catli, G., Abaci, A., and Bober, E. (2015). Maturity-onset diabetes of the young (MODY): an update. *J. Pediatr. Endocrinol. Metab.* 28: 251–263.

7. Hattersley, A.T. and Patel, K.A. (2017). Precision diabetes: learning from monogenic diabetes. *Diabetologia* 60: 769–777.

8. Naylor, R., Knight Johnson, A., and del Gaudio, D. (1993). Maturity-onset diabetes of the young overview. In *GeneReviews*®R, M.P. Adam, H.H. Ardinger, R.A. Pagon, S.E. Wallace, L.J.H. Bean, G. Mirzaa, and A. Amemiya, eds. Seattle, WA. University of Washington.

9. Loeys, B.L., Dietz, H.C., Braverman, A.C. et al. (2010). The revised Ghent nosology for the Marfan syndrome. *J. Med. Genet.* 47: 476–485.

10. Dietz, H. (1993). Marfan syndrome. In: *GeneReviews*® (ed. M.P. Adam, H.H. Ardinger, R.A. Pagon, et al.). Seattle, WA: University of Washington.

11. Roberts, A.E., Allanson, J.E., Tartaglia, M., and Gelb, B.D. (2013). Noonan syndrome. *Lancet* 381: 333–342.

12. Allanson, J.E. and Roberts, A.E. (1993). Noonan syndrome. In: *GeneReviews*® (ed. M.P. Adam, H.H. Ardinger, R.A. Pagon, et al.). Seattle, WA: University of Washington.

13. Williams, V.C., Lucas, J., Babcock, M.A. et al. (2009). Neurofibromatosis type 1 revisited. *Pediatrics* 123: 124–133.

14. Friedman, J.M. (1993). Neurofibromatosis 1. In: *GeneReviews*® (ed. M.P. Adam, H.H. Ardinger, R.A. Pagon, et al.). Seattle, WA: University of Washington.

15. Khan, S.A., Muhammad, N., Khan, M.A. et al. (2016). Genetics of human Bardet-Biedl syndrome, an updates. *Clin. Genet.* 90: 3–15.

16. Forsyth, R.L. and Gunay-Aygun, M. (1993). Bardet-Biedl Syndrome Overview. In: *GeneReviews*® (ed. M.P. Adam, H.H. Ardinger, R.A. Pagon, et al.). Seattle, WA: University of Washington.

17. Jones, K., Jones, M., and del Campo, M. (2021). *Smith's Recognizable Patterns of Human Malformation*. Philadelphia, PA: Elsevier, Inc.

18. Petrucelli, N., Daly, M.B., and Pal, T. (1993). BRCA1- and BRCA2-associated hereditary breast and ovarian cancer. In: *GeneReviews*® (ed. M.P. Adam, H.H. Ardinger, R.A. Pagon, et al.). Seattle, WA: University of Washington.

19. Kuchenbaecker, K.B., Hopper, J.L., Barnes, D.R. et al. (2017). Risks of breast, ovarian, and contralateral breast cancer for BRCA1 and BRCA2 mutation carriers. *JAMA* 317: 2402–2416.

20. Solomon, B.D. (2011). VACTERL/VATER association. *Orphanet J. Rare Dis.* 6: 56.

21. Solomon, B.D., Baker, L.A., Bear, K.A. et al. (2014). An approach to the identification of anomalies and etiologies in neonates with identified or suspected VACTERL (vertebral defects, anal atresia, tracheo-esophageal fistula with esophageal atresia, cardiac anomalies, renal anomalies, and limb anomalies) association. *J. Pediatr.* 164 (451–457): e451.

22. Solomon, B.D. (2018). The etiology of VACTERL association: current knowledge and hypotheses. *Am. J. Med. Genet. C Semin. Med. Genet.* 178: 440–446.

23. Wattendorf, D.J. and Muenke, M. (2005). Prader-Willi syndrome. *Am. Fam. Physician* 72: 827–830.

24. Driscoll, D.J., Miller, J.L., Schwartz, S., and Cassidy, S.B. (1993). Prader-Willi syndrome. In: *GeneReviews®* (ed. M.P. Adam, H.H. Ardinger, R.A. Pagon, et al.). Seattle, WA: University of Washington.

25. Rotig, A., Bourgeron, T., Chretien, D. et al. (1995). Spectrum of mitochondrial DNA rearrangements in the Pearson marrow-pancreas syndrome. *Hum. Mol. Genet.* 4: 1327–1330.

26. Chinnery, P.F. (1993). Primary mitochondrial disorders overview. In: *GeneReviews®* (ed. M.P. Adam, H.H. Ardinger, R.A. Pagon, et al.). Seattle, WA: University of Washington.

27. Binder, V., Albert, M.H., Kabus, M. et al. (2006). The genotype of the original Wiskott phenotype. *N. Engl. J. Med.* 355: 1790–1793.

28. Chandra, S., Bronicki, L., Nagaraj, C.B., and Zhang, K. (1993). WAS-related disorders. In: *GeneReviews®* (ed. M.P. Adam, H.H. Ardinger, R.A. Pagon, et al.). Seattle, WA: University of Washington.

29. Krakow, D. and Rimoin, D.L. (2010). The skeletal dysplasias. *Genet. Med.* 12: 327–341.

30. Legare, J.M. (1993). Achondroplasia. In: *GeneReviews®* (ed. M.P. Adam, H.H. Ardinger, R.A. Pagon, et al.). Seattle, WA: University of Washington.

31. Sahin, M., Henske, E.P., Manning, B.D. et al. (2016). Advances and future directions for tuberous sclerosis complex research: recommendations from the 2015 strategic planning conference. *Pediatr. Neurol.* 60: 1–12.

32. Northrup, H., Koenig, M.K., Pearson, D.A., and Au, K.S. (1993). Tuberous sclerosis complex. In: *GeneReviews®* (ed. M.P. Adam, H.H. Ardinger, R.A. Pagon, et al.). Seattle, WA: University of Washington.

33. Walker, F.O. (2007). Huntington's disease. *Lancet* 369: 218–228.

34. Caron, N.S., Wright, G.E.B., and Hayden, M.R. (1993). Huntington disease. In: *GeneReviews®* (ed. M.P. Adam, H.H. Ardinger, R.A. Pagon, et al.). Seattle, WA: University of Washington.

35. Steiner, R.D. and Basel, D. (1993). COL1A1/2 osteogenesis imperfecta. In: *GeneReviews®* (ed. M.P. Adam, H.H. Ardinger, R.A. Pagon, et al.). Seattle, WA: University of Washington.

36. Weksberg, R., Shuman, C., and Beckwith, J.B. (2010). Beckwith-Wiedemann syndrome. *Eur. J. Hum. Genet.* 18: 8–14.

37. Shuman, C., Beckwith, J.B., and Weksberg, R. (1993). Beckwith-Wiedemann syndrome. In: *GeneReviews®* (ed. M.P. Adam, H.H. Ardinger, R.A. Pagon, et al.). Seattle, WA: University of Washington.

38. Leggett, V., Jacobs, P., Nation, K. et al. (2010). Neurocognitive outcomes of individuals with a sex chromosome trisomy: XXX, XYY, or XXY: a systematic review. *Dev. Med. Child Neurol.* 52: 119–129.

39. Margari, L., Lamanna, A.L., Craig, F. et al. (2014). Autism spectrum disorders in XYY syndrome: two new cases and systematic review of the literature. *Eur. J. Pediatr.* 173: 277–283.

40. Samango-Sprouse, C., Kirkizlar, E., Hall, M.P. et al. (2016). Incidence of X and Y chromosomal aneuploidy in a large child bearing population. *PLoS One* 11: e0161045.

41. Rosendahl, J., Bodeker, H., Mossner, J., and Teich, N. (2007). Hereditary chronic pancreatitis. *Orphanet J. Rare Dis.* 2: 1.

42. Shelton, C., LaRusch, J., and Whitcomb, D.C. (1993). Pancreatitis overview. In: *GeneReviews*® (ed. M.P. Adam, H.H. Ardinger, R.A. Pagon, et al.). (Seattle, WA: University of Washington.

43. van den Hout, H.M., Hop, W., van Diggelen, O.P. et al. (2003). The natural course of infantile Pompe's disease: 20 original cases compared with 133 cases from the literature. *Pediatrics* 112: 332–340.

44. Disease, A.W.G.O.M.O.P., Kishnani, P.S., Steiner, R.D. et al. (2006). Pompe disease diagnosis and management guideline. *Genet. Med.* 8: 267–288.

45. Leslie, N. and Bailey, L. (1993). Pompe disease. In: *GeneReviews*® (ed. M.P. Adam, H.H. Ardinger, R.A. Pagon, et al.). Seattle, WA: University of Washington.

46. Cheung, E.N., George, S.R., Costain, G.A. et al. (2014). Prevalence of hypocalcaemia and its associated features in 22q11.2 deletion syndrome. *Clin. Endocrinol.* 81: 190–196.

47. McDonald-McGinn, D.M., Hain, H.S., Emanuel, B.S., and Zackai, E.H. (1993). 22q11.2 deletion syndrome. In: *GeneReviews*® (ed. M.P. Adam, H.H. Ardinger, R.A. Pagon, et al.). Seattle, WA: University of Washington.

48. Valente, E.M., Dallapiccola, B., and Bertini, E. (2013). Joubert syndrome and related disorders. *Handb. Clin. Neurol.* 113: 1879–1888.

49. Parisi, M. and Glass, I. (1993). Joubert syndrome. In: *GeneReviews*® (ed. M.P. Adam, H.H. Ardinger, R.A. Pagon, et al.). Seattle, WA: University of Washington.

50. Morris, C.A. (1993). Williams syndrome. In: *GeneReviews*® (ed. M.P. Adam, H.H. Ardinger, R.A. Pagon, et al.). Seattle, WA: University of Washington.

51. Chung, M.G. (2015). Hereditary hemorrhagic telangiectasia. *Handb. Clin. Neurol.* 132: 185–197.

52. McDonald, J. and Pyeritz, R.E. (1993). Hereditary hemorrhagic telangiectasia. In: *GeneReviews*® (ed. M.P. Adam, H.H. Ardinger, R.A. Pagon, et al.). Seattle, WA: University of Washington.

53. Schmidt, L.S. and Linehan, W.M. (2015). Molecular genetics and clinical features of Birt-Hogg-Dube syndrome. *Nat. Rev. Urol.* 12: 558–569.

54. Sattler, E.C. and Steinlein, O.K. (1993). Birt-Hogg-dube syndrome. In: *GeneReviews*® (ed. M.P. Adam, H.H. Ardinger, R.A. Pagon, et al.). Seattle, WA: University of Washington.

55. Bonkowsky, J.L., Nelson, C., Kingston, J.L. et al. (2010). The burden of inherited leukodystrophies in children. *Neurology* 75: 718–725.

56. Vanderver, A., Tonduti, D., Schiffmann, R. et al. (1993). Leukodystrophy overview – retired chapter, for historical reference only. In: *GeneReviews*® (ed. M.P. Adam, H.H. Ardinger, R.A. Pagon, et al.). Seattle, WA: University of Washington.

57. Vincent, M., Genevieve, D., Ostertag, A. et al. (2016). Treacher Collins syndrome: a clinical and molecular study based on a large series of patients. *Genet. Med.* 18: 49–56.

58. Katsanis, S.H. and Jabs, E.W. (1993). Treacher collins syndrome. In: *GeneReviews*® (ed. M.P. Adam, H.H. Ardinger, R.A. Pagon, et al.). Seattle, WA: University of Washington.

59. Hassett, S., Smith, G.H., and Holland, A.J. (2012). Prune belly syndrome. *Pediatr. Surg. Int.* 28: 219–228.

60. Stevenson, R.E., Allanson, J.G., Everman, D.B., and Solomon, B.D. (2016). *Human Malformations and Related Anomalies*. New York: OxfordUniversity Press).

61. Twigg, S.R., Kan, R., Babbs, C. et al. (2004). Mutations of ephrin-B1 (EFNB1), a marker of tissue boundary formation, cause craniofrontonasal syndrome. *Proc. Natl. Acad. Sci. U. S. A.* 101: 8652–8657.

62. Twigg, S.R., Babbs, C., van den Elzen, M.E. et al. (2013). Cellular interference in craniofrontonasal syndrome: males mosaic for mutations in the X-linked EFNB1 gene are more severely affected than true hemizygotes. *Hum. Mol. Genet.* 22: 1654–1662.

63. Bergman, J.E., Janssen, N., Hoefsloot, L.H. et al. (2011). CHD7 mutations and CHARGE syndrome: the clinical implications of an expanding phenotype. *J. Med. Genet.* 48: 334–342.

64. van Ravenswaaij-Arts, C.M., Hefner, M., Blake, K., and Martin, D.M. (1993). CHD7 disorder. In: *GeneReviews®* (ed. M.P. Adam, H.H. Ardinger, R.A. Pagon, et al.). Seattle, WA: University of Washington.

65. Hildebrandt, F., Benzing, T., and Katsanis, N. (2011). Ciliopathies. *N. Engl. J. Med.* 364: 1533–1543.

66. Reiter, J.F. and Leroux, M.R. (2017). Genes and molecular pathways underpinning ciliopathies. *Nat. Rev. Mol. Cell Biol.* 18: 533–547.

67. Kaler, S.G. (2013). Inborn errors of copper metabolism. *Handb. Clin. Neurol.* 113: 1745–1754.

68. Ferreira, C.R. and Gahl, W.A. (2017). Disorders of metal metabolism. *Transl Sci Rare Dis* 2: 101–139.

69. Saleh, M., Kamath, B.M., and Chitayat, D. (2016). Alagille syndrome: clinical perspectives. *Appl. Clin. Genet.* 9: 75–82.

70. Spinner, N.B., Gilbert, M.A., Loomes, K.M., and Krantz, I.D. (1993). Alagille syndrome. In: *GeneReviews®* (ed. M.P. Adam, H.H. Ardinger, R.A. Pagon, et al.). Seattle, WA: University of Washington.

71. Evans, D.G. and Farndon, P.A. (1993). Nevoid basal cell carcinoma syndrome. In: *GeneReviews®* (ed. M.P. Adam, H.H. Ardinger, R.A. Pagon, et al.). Seattle, WA: University of Washington.

72. Carlyle, B.E., Borowitz, D.S., and Glick, P.L. (2012). A review of pathophysiology and management of fetuses and neonates with meconium ileus for the pediatric surgeon. *J. Pediatr. Surg.* 47: 772–781.

73. Ong, T., Marshall, S.G., Karczeski, B.A. et al. (1993). Cystic fibrosis and congenital absence of the vas deferens. In: *GeneReviews®* (ed. M.P. Adam, H.H. Ardinger, R.A. Pagon, et al.). Seattle, WA: University of Washington.

74. Half, E., Bercovich, D., and Rozen, P. (2009). Familial adenomatous polyposis. *Orphanet J. Rare Dis.* 4: 22.

75. Jasperson, K.W., Patel, S.G., and Ahnen, D.J. (1993). APC-associated polyposis conditions. In: *GeneReviews®* (ed. M.P. Adam, H.H. Ardinger, R.A. Pagon, et al.). (Seattle, WA: University of Washington.

76. Rogers, R.C. and Abidi, F.E. (1993). Coffin-Lowry syndrome. In: *GeneReviews®* (ed. M.P. Adam, H.H. Ardinger, R.A. Pagon, et al.). Seattle, WA: University of Washington.

77. Robin, N.H., Moran, R.T., and Ala-Kokko, L. (1993). Stickler syndrome. In: *GeneReviews®* (ed. M.P. Adam, H.H. Ardinger, R.A. Pagon, et al.). Seattle, WA: University of Washington.

78. Bird, T.D. (1993). Charcot-Marie-Tooth (CMT) hereditary neuropathy overview. In: *GeneReviews®* (ed. M.P. Adam, H.H. Ardinger, R.A. Pagon, et al.). Seattle, WA: University of Washington.

79. Bergstrom, S., Carr, H., Petersson, G. et al. (2016). Trends in congenital heart defects in infants with Down syndrome. *Pediatrics* 138: 1–9.

80. Diogenes, T.C.P., Mourato, F.A., de Lima Filho, J.L., and Mattos, S.D.S. (2017). Gender differences in the prevalence of congenital heart disease in Down's syndrome: a brief meta-analysis. *BMC Med. Genet.* 18: 111.

81. Maher, E.R., Neumann, H.P., and Richard, S. (2011). von Hippel-Lindau disease: a clinical and scientific review. *Eur. J. Hum. Genet.* 19: 617–623.

82. van Leeuwaarde, R.S., Ahmad, S., Links, T.P., and Giles, R.H. (1993). Von Hippel-Lindau syndrome. In: *GeneReviews®* (ed. M.P. Adam, H.H. Ardinger, R.A. Pagon, et al.). Seattle, WA: University of Washington.

83. Dobyns, W.B., Reiner, O., Carrozzo, R., and Ledbetter, D.H. (1993). Lissencephaly. A human brain malformation associated with deletion of the LIS1 gene located at chromosome 17p13. *JAMA* 270: 2838–2842.

84. Da Costa, L., O'Donohue, M.F., van Dooijeweert, B. et al. (2018). Molecular approaches to diagnose Diamond-Blackfan anemia: the EuroDBA experience. *Eur. J. Med. Genet.* 61: 664–673.

85. Sieff, C. (1993). Diamond-Blackfan anemia. In: *GeneReviews®* (ed. M.P. Adam, H.H. Ardinger, R.A. Pagon, et al.). Seattle, WA: University of Washington.

86. Brugada, R., Campuzano, O., Sarquella-Brugada, G. et al. (1993). Brugada syndrome. In: *GeneReviews®* (ed. M.P. Adam, H.H. Ardinger, R.A. Pagon, et al.). Seattle, WA: University of Washington.

87. Hosseini, S.M., Kim, R., Udupa, S. et al. (2018). Reappraisal of reported genes for sudden arrhythmic death: evidence-based evaluation of gene validity for Brugada syndrome. *Circulation* 138: 1195–1205.

88. Fernandez Garcia, M.S. and Teruya-Feldstein, J. (2014). The diagnosis and treatment of dyskeratosis congenita: a review. *J. Blood Med.* 5: 157–167.

89. Savage, S.A. (1993). Dyskeratosis congenita. In: *GeneReviews®* (ed. M.P. Adam, H.H. Ardinger, R.A. Pagon, et al.). Seattle, WA: University of Washington.

90. Kashtan, C.E. (1999). Alport syndrome. An inherited disorder of renal, ocular, and cochlear basement membranes. *Medicine* 78: 338–360.

91. Kashtan, C.E. (1993). Alport syndrome. In: *GeneReviews®* (ed. M.P. Adam, H.H. Ardinger, R.A. Pagon, et al.). Seattle, WA: University of Washington.

92. Eng, C. (1993). Multiple endocrine neoplasia type 2. In: *GeneReviews®* (ed. M.P. Adam, H.H. Ardinger, R.A. Pagon, et al.). Seattle, WA: University of Washington.

93. Dagli, A.I., Mathews, J., and Williams, C.A. (1993). Angelman syndrome. In: *GeneReviews®* (ed. M.P. Adam, H.H. Ardinger, R.A. Pagon, et al.). Seattle, WA: University of Washington.

94. Altschwager, P., Ambrosio, L., Swanson, E.A. et al. (2017). Juvenile macular degenerations. *Semin. Pediatr. Neurol.* 24: 104–109.

95. Tanna, P., Strauss, R.W., Fujinami, K., and Michaelides, M. (2017). Stargardt disease: clinical features, molecular genetics, animal models and therapeutic options. *Br. J. Ophthalmol.* 101: 25–30.

96. Fischbach, B.V., Trout, K.L., Lewis, J. et al. (2005). WAGR syndrome: a clinical review of 54 cases. *Pediatrics* 116: 984–988.

Chapter 3

97. Moosajee, M., Hingorani, M., and Moore, A.T. (1993). PAX6-related aniridia. In: *GeneReviews*® (ed. M.P. Adam, H.H. Ardinger, R.A. Pagon, et al.). Seattle, WA: University of Washington.

98. Russell, M.B. and Ducros, A. (2011). Sporadic and familial hemiplegic migraine: pathophysiological mechanisms, clinical characteristics, diagnosis, and management. *Lancet Neurol.* 10: 457–470.

99. Jen, J.C. (1993). Familial hemiplegic migraine. In: *GeneReviews*® (ed. M.P. Adam, H.H. Ardinger, R.A. Pagon, et al.). Seattle, WA: University of Washington.

100. Gower, W.A. and Nogee, L.M. (2011). Surfactant dysfunction. *Paediatr. Respir. Rev.* 12: 223–229.

101. Turcu, S., Ashton, E., Jenkins, L. et al. (2013). Genetic testing in children with surfactant dysfunction. *Arch. Dis. Child.* 98: 490–495.

102. Lucas, J.S., Burgess, A., Mitchison, H.M. et al. (2014). Diagnosis and management of primary ciliary dyskinesia. *Arch. Dis. Child.* 99: 850–856.

103. Mirra, V., Werner, C., and Santamaria, F. (2017). Primary ciliary dyskinesia: an update on clinical aspects, genetics, diagnosis, and future treatment strategies. *Front. Pediatr.* 5: 135.

104. Zariwala, M.A., Knowles, M.R., and Leigh, M.W. (1993). Primary ciliary dyskinesia. In: *GeneReviews*® (ed. M.P. Adam, H.H. Ardinger, R.A. Pagon, et al.). Seattle, WA: University of Washington.

105. Wong, B.K.Y. and Sutton, V.R. (2018). Aicardi syndrome, an unsolved mystery: review of diagnostic features, previous attempts, and future opportunities for genetic examination. *Am. J. Med. Genet. C Semin. Med. Genet.* 178: 423–431.

106. Sutton, V.R. and Van den Veyver, I.B. (1993). Aicardi syndrome. In: *GeneReviews*® (ed. M.P. Adam, H.H. Ardinger, R.A. Pagon, et al.). Seattle, WA: University of Washington.

107. Fridovich-Keil, J.L., Gubbels, C.S., Spencer, J.B. et al. (2011). Ovarian function in girls and women with GALT-deficiency galactosemia. *J. Inherit. Metab. Dis.* 34: 357–366.

108. Berry, G.T. (1993). Classic galactosemia and clinical variant galactosemia. In: *GeneReviews*® (ed. M.P. Adam, H.H. Ardinger, R.A. Pagon, et al.). Seattle, WA: University of Washington.

109. Misago, N. and Narisawa, Y. (2000). Sebaceous neoplasms in Muir-Torre syndrome. *Am. J. Dermatopathol.* 22: 155–161.

110. South, C.D., Hampel, H., Comeras, I. et al. (2008). The frequency of Muir-Torre syndrome among Lynch syndrome families. *J. Natl. Cancer Inst.* 100: 277–281.

111. Idos, G. and Valle, L. (1993). Lynch syndrome. In: *GeneReviews*® (ed. M.P. Adam, H.H. Ardinger, R.A. Pagon, et al.). Seattle, WA: University of Washington.

112. Parisi, M.A. (1993). Hirschsprung disease overview – retired chapter, for historical reference only. In: *GeneReviews*® (ed. M.P. Adam, H.H. Ardinger, R.A. Pagon, et al.). Seattle, WA: University of Washington.

113. Leebeek, F.W. and Eikenboom, J.C. (2016). Von Willebrand's disease. *N. Engl. J. Med.* 375: 2067–2080.

114. Swami, A. and Kaur, V. (2017). von Willebrand disease: a concise review and update for the practicing physician. *Clin. Appl. Thromb. Hemost.* 23: 900–910.

Chapter 3

115. Zenker, M., Aigner, T., Wendler, O. et al. (2004). Human laminin beta2 deficiency causes congenital nephrosis with mesangial sclerosis and distinct eye abnormalities. *Hum. Mol. Genet.* 13: 2625–2632.

116. Matejas, V., Hinkes, B., Alkandari, F. et al. (2010). Mutations in the human laminin beta2 (LAMB2) gene and the associated phenotypic spectrum. *Hum. Mutat.* 31: 992–1002.

117. Jadeja, S., Smyth, I., Pitera, J.E. et al. (2005). Identification of a new gene mutated in Fraser syndrome and mouse myelencephalic blebs. *Nat. Genet.* 37: 520–525.

118. Tessier, A., Sarreau, M., Pelluard, F. et al. (2016). Fraser syndrome: features suggestive of prenatal diagnosis in a review of 38 cases. *Prenat. Diagn.* 36: 1270–1275.

119. Ferreira, C.R. and Gahl, W.A. (2017). Lysosomal storage diseases. *Transl. Sci. Rare Dis.* 2: 1–71.

120. Mehta, A. and Hughes, D.A. (1993). Fabry disease. In: *GeneReviews®* (ed. M.P. Adam, H.H. Ardinger, R.A. Pagon, et al.). Seattle, WA: University of Washington.

121. Wanner, C., Arad, M., Baron, R. et al. (2018). European expert consensus statement on therapeutic goals in Fabry disease. *Mol. Genet. Metab.* 124: 189–203.

122. Baser, M.E., Friedman, J.M., Aeschliman, D. et al. (2002). Predictors of the risk of mortality in neurofibromatosis 2. *Am. J. Hum. Genet.* 71: 715–723.

123. Evans, D.G. (1993). Neurofibromatosis 2. In: *GeneReviews®* (ed. M.P. Adam, H.H. Ardinger, R.A. Pagon, et al.). (Seattle, WA.

124. Zamel, R., Khan, R., Pollex, R.L., and Hegele, R.A. (2008). Abetalipoproteinemia: two case reports and literature review. *Orphanet J. Rare Dis.* 3: 19.

125. Jung, H.H., Danek, A., and Walker, R.H. (2011). Neuroacanthocytosis syndromes. *Orphanet J. Rare Dis.* 6: 68.

126. Lee, J. and Hegele, R.A. (2014). Abetalipoproteinemia and homozygous hypobetalipoproteinemia: a framework for diagnosis and management. *J. Inherit. Metab. Dis.* 37: 333–339.

127. Burnett, J.R., Hooper, A.J., and Hegele, R.A. (1993). Abetalipoproteinemia. In: *GeneReviews®* (ed. M.P. Adam, H.H. Ardinger, R.A. Pagon, et al.). Seattle, WA: University of Washington.

128. Yu-Wai-Man, P. and Chinnery, P.F. (1993). Leber hereditary optic neuropathy. In: *GeneReviews®* (ed. M.P. Adam, H.H. Ardinger, R.A. Pagon, et al.). Seattle, WA: University of Washington.

129. Kohlhase, J. (1993). Townes-Brocks syndrome. In: *GeneReviews®* (ed. M.P. Adam, H.H. Ardinger, R.A. Pagon, et al.). Seattle, WA: University of Washington.

130. Bozal-Basterra, L., Martin-Ruiz, I., Pirone, L. et al. (2018). Truncated SALL1 impedes primary cilia function in Townes-Brocks syndrome. *Am. J. Hum. Genet.* 102: 249–265.

131. Wang, M.M. (2018). Cadasil. *Handb. Clin. Neurol.* 148: 733–743.

132. Hack, R.J., Rutten, J., and Lesnik Oberstein, S.A.J. (1993). Cadasil. In: *GeneReviews®* (ed. M.P. Adam, H.H. Ardinger, R.A. Pagon, et al.). Seattle, WA: University of Washington.

133. Harris, P.C. and Torres, V.E. (1993). Polycystic kidney disease, autosomal dominant. In: *GeneReviews®* (ed. M.P. Adam, H.H. Ardinger, R.A. Pagon, et al.). Seattle, WA: University of Washington.
134. Bergmann, C., Guay-Woodford, L.M., Harris, P.C. et al. (2018). Polycystic kidney disease. *Nat. Rev. Dis. Primers.* 4: 50.
135. Fard, M.A., Wu-Chen, W.Y., Man, B.L., and Miller, N.R. (2010). Septo-optic dysplasia. *Pediatr. Endocrinol. Rev.* 8: 18–24.
136. Sataite, I., Cudlip, S., Jayamohan, J., and Ganau, M. (2021). Septo-optic dysplasia. *Handb. Clin. Neurol.* 181: 51–64.
137. Sweeney, W.E. and Avner, E.D. (1993). Polycystic kidney disease, autosomal recessive. In: *GeneReviews®* (ed. M.P. Adam, H.H. Ardinger, R.A. Pagon, et al.). Seattle, WA: University of Washington.
138. Klein, C., Lohmann, K., Marras, C., and Munchau, A. (1993). Hereditary dystonia overview. In: *GeneReviews®* (ed. M.P. Adam, H.H. Ardinger, R.A. Pagon, et al.). Seattle, WA: University of Washington.
139. Newby, R.E., Thorpe, D.E., Kempster, P.A., and Alty, J.E. (2017). A history of dystonia: ancient to modern. *Mov. Disord. Clin. Pract.* 4: 478–485.
140. Meijer, I.A. and Pearson, T.S. (2018). The twists of pediatric dystonia: phenomenology, classification, and genetics. *Semin. Pediatr. Neurol.* 25: 65–74.
141. El-Chemaly, S. and Young, L.R. (2016). Hermansky-Pudlak syndrome. *Clin. Chest Med.* 37: 505–511.
142. Vicary, G.W., Vergne, Y., Santiago-Cornier, A. et al. (2016). Pulmonary fibrosis in Hermansky-Pudlak syndrome. *Ann. Am. Thorac. Soc.* 13: 1839–1846.
143. Huizing, M., Malicdan, M.C.V., Gochuico, B.R., and Gahl, W.A. (1993). Hermansky-Pudlak syndrome. In: *GeneReviews®* (ed. M.P. Adam, H.H. Ardinger, R.A. Pagon, et al.). Seattle, WA: University of Washington.
144. Gatti, R. and Perlman, S. (1993). Ataxia-telangiectasia. In: *GeneReviews®* (ed. M.P. Adam, H.H. Ardinger, R.A. Pagon, et al.). Seattle, WA: University of Washington.
145. Rothblum-Oviatt, C., Wright, J., Lefton-Greif, M.A. et al. (2016). Ataxia telangiectasia: a review. *Orphanet J. Rare Dis.* 11: 159.
146. Cochat, P. and Rumsby, G. (2013). Primary hyperoxaluria. *N. Engl. J. Med.* 369: 649–658.
147. Ben-Shalom, E. and Frishberg, Y. (2015). Primary hyperoxalurias: diagnosis and treatment. *Pediatr. Nephrol.* 30: 1781–1791.
148. Nyberg, D.A., Mack, L.A., Hirsch, J., and Mahony, B.S. (1988). Abnormalities of fetal cranial contour in sonographic detection of spina bifida: evaluation of the "lemon" sign. *Radiology* 167: 387–392.
149. Van den Hof, M.C., Nicolaides, K.H., Campbell, J., and Campbell, S. (1990). Evaluation of the lemon and banana signs in one hundred thirty fetuses with open spina bifida. *Am. J. Obstet. Gynecol.* 162: 322–327.
150. Thomas, M. (2003). The lemon sign. *Radiology* 228: 206–207.
151. Bokenkamp, A. and Ludwig, M. (2016). The oculocerebrorenal syndrome of Lowe: an update. *Pediatr. Nephrol.* 31: 2201–2212.
152. Lewis, R.A., Nussbaum, R.L., and Brewer, E.D. (1993). Lowe syndrome. In: *GeneReviews®* (ed. M.P. Adam, H.H. Ardinger, R.A. Pagon, et al.). Seattle, WA: University of Washington.

Chapter 3

153. Nelson, A. and Myers, K. (1993). Shwachman-Diamond syndrome. In: *GeneReviews®* (ed. M.P. Adam, H.H. Ardinger, R.A. Pagon, et al.). Seattle, WA: University of Washington.

154. Nelson, A.S. and Myers, K.C. (2018). Diagnosis, treatment, and molecular pathology of Shwachman-Diamond syndrome. *Hematol. Oncol. Clin. North Am.* 32: 687–700.

155. Krow-Lucal, E.R., de Andrade, M.R., Cananea, J.N.A. et al. (2018). Association and birth prevalence of microcephaly attributable to Zika virus infection among infants in Paraiba, Brazil, in 2015–16: a case-control study. *Lancet Child Adolesc. Health* 2: 205–213.

156. Pomar, L., Vouga, M., Lambert, V. et al. (2018). Maternal-fetal transmission and adverse perinatal outcomes in pregnant women infected with Zika virus: prospective cohort study in French Guiana. *BMJ* 363: k4431.

157. Musso, D., Ko, A.I., and Baud, D. (2019). Zika virus infection – after the pandemic. *N. Engl. J. Med.* 381: 1444–1457.

158. Vester, M.E., Bilo, R.A., Karst, W.A. et al. (2015). Subdural hematomas: glutaric aciduria type 1 or abusive head trauma? A systematic review. *Forensic Sci. Med. Pathol.* 11: 405–415.

159. Vester, M.E., Visser, G., Wijburg, F.A. et al. (2016). Occurrence of subdural hematomas in Dutch glutaric aciduria type 1 patients. *Eur. J. Pediatr.* 175: 1001–1006.

160. Larson, A. and Goodman, S. (1993). Glutaric acidemia type 1. In: *GeneReviews®* (ed. M.P. Adam, H.H. Ardinger, R.A. Pagon, et al.). Seattle, WA: University of Washington.

161. Bagni, C., Tassone, F., Neri, G., and Hagerman, R. (2012). Fragile X syndrome: causes, diagnosis, mechanisms, and therapeutics. *J. Clin. Invest.* 122: 4314–4322.

162. Hunter, J.E., Berry-Kravis, E., Hipp, H., and Todd, P.K. (1993). FMR1 disorders. In: *GeneReviews®* (ed. M.P. Adam, H.H. Ardinger, R.A. Pagon, et al.). Seattle, WA: University of Washington.

163. Lewis, R.A. (1993). Oculocutaneous albinism type 1 – retired chapter, for historical reference only. In: *GeneReviews®* (ed. M.P. Adam, H.H. Ardinger, R.A. Pagon, et al.). Seattle, WA: University of Washington.

164. Kondo, H. (2018). Foveal hypoplasia and optical coherence tomographic imaging. *Taiwan J. Ophthalmol.* 8: 181–188.

165. Brady, R.O., Filling-Katz, M.R., Barton, N.W., and Pentchev, P.G. (1989). Niemann-Pick disease types C and D. *Neurol. Clin.* 7: 75–88.

166. Schuchman, E.H. and Desnick, R.J. (2017). Types A and B Niemann-Pick disease. *Mol. Genet. Metab.* 120: 27–33.

167. Tranebjaerg, L., Barrett, T., and Rendtorff, N.D. (1993). WFS1 Wolfram syndrome spectrum disorder. In: *GeneReviews®* (ed. M.P. Adam, H.H. Ardinger, R.A. Pagon, et al.). Seattle, WA: University of Washington.

168. Fahim, A.T., Daiger, S.P., and Weleber, R.G. (1993). Nonsyndromic retinitis pigmentosa overview. In *GeneReviews®*, M.P. Adam, H.H. Ardinger, R.A. Pagon, S.E. Wallace, L.J.H. Bean, G. Mirzaa, and A. Amemiya, eds. Seattle, WA. University of Washington.

Causes of Genetic Conditions and Laboratory and Testing Approaches

4

4.1. Pathogenic variants in which gene are most associated with Hereditary diffuse gastric cancer?
A. *APC*
B. *BRCA1*
C. *CDH1*
D. *EPCAM*

4.2. A woman undergoes genetic testing because of her family history. She is found to have an *FMR1* allele with 120 trinucleotide repeats. Which of the following best describes this allele?
A. Normal allele
B. Intermediate allele
C. Premutation allele
D. Full mutation allele

4.3. Which condition is often diagnosed by methods that detect abnormal neutrophil superoxide production?
A. Chediak-Higashi syndrome
B. Chronic granulomatous disease
C. Hyper IgE syndrome
D. Severe combined immunodeficiency

4.4. Based on medical history and examination, a patient is suspected to have Pallister-Killian syndrome. What tissue source(s) or sample type(s) would likely be most helpful to confirm the diagnosis?
A. CSF
B. Peripheral blood or saliva
C. Buccal swab or skin biopsy
D. Urine

4.5. Germline pathogenic variants in which gene are most commonly implicated in prostate cancer?
A. *ATM*
B. *BRCA1*
C. *BRCA2*
D. *PMS2*

4.6. Due to family history and genetic testing in affected relatives, a healthy individual is suspected to have a balanced translocation. Which test would be most likely to help efficiently identify this translocation?
A. Karyotype
B. NGS-based panel testing
C. Sanger sequencing
D. SNP-based microarray

4.7. Which choice below describes the most common pathogenic allele for Alpha-1 antitrypsin deficiency (AATD)?
A. PI*M
B. PI*Z
C. SERPINA1
D. p.Phe508del

Medical Genetics and Genomics: Questions for Board Review, First Edition. Benjamin D. Solomon.
© 2023 John Wiley & Sons Ltd. Published 2023 by John Wiley & Sons Ltd.

4.8. A patient has features consistent with Noonan syndrome. If this is the correct diagnosis, which gene is most likely to be involved?

A. *KRAS*

B. *NF1*

C. *PTPN11*

D. *RAF1*

4.9. Based on medical history and physical examination, a patient has a high suspicion of a certain diagnosis. For which of the following conditions would a more specific/targeted test (versus exome or genome sequencing) be most likely to be useful for making the molecular diagnosis?

A. Bardet-Biedl syndrome

B. Diamond-Blackfan anemia

C. Prader-Willi syndrome

D. Retinitis pigmentosa

4.10. Dravet syndrome is an infantile-onset genetic epileptic encephalopathy. What gene is most commonly involved in this condition?

A. *PCDH19*

B. *SCN1A*

C. *SCN2A*

D. *SLC2A1*

4.11. Which of the following conditions is NOT currently included in US newborn screening?

A. Alkaptonuria

B. Biotinidase deficiency

C. Congenital hypothyroidism

D. Phenylketonuria

4.12. Pathogenic variants in which gene would be suspected in a family with a history of osteosarcoma, adrenocortical carcinoma, and early-onset breast cancer?

A. *PTEN*

B. *TP53*

C. *TP63*

D. *VHL*

4.13. Familial Creutzfeldt-Jakob disease, Gerstmann-Sträussler-Scheinker (GSS) syndrome, and Fatal familial insomnia are all considered what type of genetic disorder?

A. Carnitine metabolism disorders

B. Mucopolysaccharidoses

C. Genetic prion disorders

D. Thyroidogenesis disorders

4.14. What gene is involved in Sturge-Weber syndrome and "port-wine stains"?

A. *AKT1*

B. *GNAQ*

C. *HRAS*

D. *RASA1*

4.15. What syndrome can result from a microdeletion of chromosome 5q35 or a pathogenic variant in the gene *NSD1*?

A. Miller-Dieker syndrome

B. Pallister-Killian syndrome

C. Smith-Magenis syndrome

D. Sotos syndrome

4.16. Repeat expansion in what gene is associated with Amyotrophic lateral sclerosis and Frontotemporal lobar degeneration?

A. *ATXN1*

B. *C9ORF72*

C. *FMR1*

D. *HTT*

4.17. Which condition can be associated with low TREC concentration on newborn screening?

A. Congenital hypothyroidism

B. Galactosemia

C. Phenylketonuria

D. Severe combined immunodeficiency

4.18. Colorectal cancer associated with what gene involves autosomal recessive inheritance?
A. *EPCAM*
B. *MSH2*
C. *MUTYH*
D. *PMS2*

4.19. Sickle cell disease results from the presence of at least one of what allele (along with another pathogenic variant)?
A. β+-thalassemia
B. Hemoglobin C
C. Hemoglobin D
D. Hemoglobin S

Chapter 4

4.20. A pathogenic variant in which of the following genes can cause a phenotype similar to heterozygous deletion of chromosome 17p11.2?
A. *NF1*
B. *RAI1*
C. *RBM8A*
D. *TBX1*

4.21. A two-year-old girl had normal early development, but now has developmental regression. What gene might be suspected to be involved?
A. *ATP7A*
B. *GJB2*
C. *MECP2*
D. *PAX3*

4.22. Acrodermatitis enteropathica, Birk-Landau-Perez syndrome, and Spondylocheirodysplastic Ehlers-Danlos syndrome are genetic conditions that all involve abnormalities related to metabolism of what metal?
A. Copper
B. Iron
C. Magnesium
D. Zinc

4.23. What gene might be suspected in a child with spotty lip pigmentation and a family history of GI polyps?
A. *APC*
B. *BRCA1*
C. *PMS2*
D. *STK11*

4.24. Pathogenic variants in the *ABCD1* gene can result in what X-linked condition?
A. Adrenoleukodystrophy
B. Color blindness
C. G6PD deficiency
D. Lesch-Nyhan syndrome

4.25. A male fetus has hydrocephalus due to aqueductal stenosis. A pathogenic variant in which gene might be suspected?
A. *ACTB*
B. *CASK*
C. *L1CAM*
D. *RELN*

4.26. In Hereditary hemochromatosis due to pathogenic variants in the HFE gene, which of the following variants is relatively common in non-Hispanic white individuals?
A. c.35delG
B. Monosomy X
C. p.Cys282Tyr
D. p.Pro250Arg

4.27. A variant identified through genetic testing has been reclassified – it was originally considered to be a variant of uncertain significance (VUS) and is now considered to be likely pathogenic. What type of data could have contributed to this change in variant classification?
A. Functional
B. Population
C. Segregation
D. All of the above

4.28. A patient has pleuropulmonary blastoma and a personal and has a family history of other tumor types. What gene is most likely to be involved?

A. *APC* C. *MYH6*
B. *DICER1* D. *RET*

4.29. Gaucher disease results from deficiency of what enzyme?

A. Alpha-glucosidase C. Galactocerebrosidase
B. Arylsulfatase A D. Glucocerebrosidase

4.30. An infant girl had neonatal skin blistering and "warts" on her limbs a few months later. What gene might be suspected?

A. *IKBKG* C. *PTCH1*
B. *NF1* D. *TSC1*

4.31. An infant has a positive newborn screen for X-linked adrenoleukodystrophy (X-ALD). Follow-up tests are negative for X-ALD, but the child starts to show signs of developmental delay in infancy. What condition should be considered?

A. Aarskog syndrome C. Alagille syndrome
B. Aicardi-Goutières syndrome D. Alpha thalassemia

4.32. Genetic testing related to which Lynch syndrome gene can be complicated by the presence of pseudogenes?

A. *MLH1* C. *MSH6*
B. *MSH2* D. *PMS2*

4.33. Cardiac amyloidosis due to the p.Val122Ile variant in the *TTR* gene is more prevalent in individuals of what ancestry?

A. African C. Middle Eastern
B. Asian D. Northern European

4.34. Pathogenic variants in which gene result in Legius syndrome?

A. *NF1* C. *SPRED1*
B. *NF2* D. *TSC1*

4.35. A patient has prenatal-onset growth deficiency, mild immunodeficiency, photosensitivity, and increased cancer risk. Laboratory testing shows increased sister chromatid exchange. What condition is most likely?

A. Ataxia-telangiectasia C. Fanconi anemia
B. Bloom syndrome D. Werner syndrome

4.36. Based on current evidence, germline pathogenic variants in which gene account for the highest proportion of cases of familial malignant melanoma?

A. *APC* C. *CDKN2A*
B. *BAP1* D. *MSH2*

4.37. A patient is suspected to have mosaicism for a specific genetic variant (a rare single nucleotide variant). Which of the following assays would likely provide the most precise information about the level of mosaicism for this variant?

A. Droplet digital PCR C. SNP microarray
B. Genome sequencing D. NGS-based panel testing

4.38. Trinucleotide repeat expansions affecting what gene result in Myotonic dystrophy type 1?

A. *DMPK* C. *FXN*
B. *FMR1* D. *HTT*

4.39. Genetic causes of hypertrophic cardiomyopathy frequently involve pathogenic variants that cause dysfunction of what structure?
A. Distal tubule
B. Lysosome
C. Ribosome
D. Sarcomere

4.40. A patient and her father have a history of multiple benign bone tumors, identified as osteochondromas. Which genes are involved in this condition?
A. *EXT1, EXT2*
B. *FGFR1, FGFR2, FGFR3*
C. *NF1, NF2*
D. *ZIC2, ZIC3*

Chapter 4

4.41. Researchers are studying potential genetic contributions to a common condition. They use a genome-wide SNP array to examine thousands of people with and without the condition to see which variants correlate with the condition's presence. Which best describes this approach?
A. GWAS
B. Karyotype
C. Linkage analysis
D. RNA-Seq

4.42. In most populations, pathogenic variants in what gene are the most common cause of severe-to-profound autosomal recessive nonsyndromic hearing loss?
A. *COL11A2*
B. *GJB2*
C. *GJB6*
D. *MITF*

4.43. Which pathogenic variant (mutation) is most common in Spinal muscular atrophy related to the *SMN1* gene?
A. c.1138G>A
B. Deletion 22q11.2
C. Exon 8 (old literature: exon 7) loss
D. Triploidy or trisomy

4.44. Pathogenic variants in what gene cause Hutchinson-Gilford progeria syndrome?
A. *ABCA1*
B. *FLNA*
C. *LMNA*
D. *PHEX*

4.45. Laboratory testing that shows elevated very long-chain fatty acids (VLCFA) would be most suggestive of which category of disorder?
A. Peroxisomal
B. Urea cycle
C. Mitochondrial
D. Lysosomal storage

4.46. Pathogenic variants in what gene cause Nijmegen breakage syndrome in the biallelic (homozygous or compound heterozygous) state and can involve increased risk of breast cancer, prostate cancer, as well as other malignancies, in the heterozygous state?
A. *MSH2*
B. *NBN*
C. *NF1*
D. *TP53*

4.47. Which acylcarnitine is elevated (e.g. on newborn screening) in conditions including Ethylmalonic encephalopathy, Multiple acyl CoA dehydrogenase deficiency, Glutaric acidemia types IIA, IIB, and IIC, Isobutyryl CoA dehydrogenase deficiency, and Short-chain Acyl CoA dehydrogenase deficiency?
A. C0
B. C3
C. C4
D. C99

4.48. Somatic activating pathogenic variants in what gene can cause McCune-Albright syndrome?
A. *GNAS*
B. *NF2*
C. *SPRED1*
D. *VHL*

4.49. Fetal exposure to what agent would be most likely to cause facial asymmetry, microtia, and cardiovascular and brain anomalies?

A. Isotretinoin

B. Methotrexate

C. Valproate

D. Warfarin

4.50. Alpers-Huttenlocher syndrome, Kearns-Sayre syndrome, Leigh syndrome, MELAS, and MERRF are all conditions that cause disease primarily related to effects on which of the following organelles or cell types?

A. Lysosome

B. Mitochondria

C. Neutrophil

D. Peroxisome

4.51. A patient has a family history that is highly suspicious for Brugada syndrome. Assuming the clinical suspicion is correct, what gene is most likely to be involved?

A. *CACNA1C*

B. *SCN1B*

C. *SCN5A*

D. *SEMA3A*

4.52. Which karyotype result would correspond to a clinical diagnosis of Klinefelter syndrome?

A. 45,X

B. 47,XXX

C. 47,XXY

D. 47,XYY

4.53. Deficiency of what enzyme is the most common cause of Congenital adrenal hyperplasia?

A. 21-hydroxylase

B. Arylsulfatase A

C. Beta-glucosidase

D. Glucocerebrosidase

4.54. Pathogenic variants in what gene(s) would be most likely suspected in a child with an atypical teratoid/rhabdoid tumor (ATRT)?

A. *APC*

B. *BRCA1, BRCA2*

C. *SMARCA4, SMARCB1*

D. *TSC1, TSC2*

4.55. Pathogenic variants in what gene cause Grieg cephalopolysyndactyly and Pallister-Hall syndromes?

A. *GLI1*

B. *GLI2*

C. *GLI3*

D. *SIX6*

4.56. About what percent of fetuses with cystic hygroma will have a major cytogenomic (chromosomal) anomaly, identifiable by karyotype?

A. 1%

B. 10%

C. 50%

D. 97%

4.57. Pathogenic variants (mutations) in what gene result in Mowat-Wilson syndrome?

A. *WNT5A*

B. *XIAP*

C. *YARS*

D. *ZEB2*

4.58. A patient and his brother both have pathogenic variants in the gene *AVPR2* and have a history of failure to thrive with polyuria and polydipsia; their serum sodium levels were elevated prior to treatment. What condition do they have?

A. Diabetes insipidus

B. Diabetes mellitus

C. Fanconi syndrome

D. Polycystic kidney disease

4.59. Severe deficiency of the enzyme hypoxanthine-guanine phosophoribosyltrans-ferase results in what X-linked condition that includes intellectual disability (with self-injurious behavior) and uric acid overproduction?
    A. Alkaptonuria
    B. Biotinidase deficiency
    C. Hypophosphotasia
    D. Lesch-Nyhan syndrome

4.60. Pathogenic variants in what gene are most frequently associated with Congenital central hypoventilation syndrome?
    A. *C9ORF72*
    B. *PHOX2B*
    C. *PMP22*
    D. *TPP1*

Chapter 4

4.61. A neonate has nasal hypoplasia and skeletal anomalies (stippled vertebrae and bony epiphyses). In utero exposure to what agent might be suspected?
    A. Alcohol
    B. Cytomegalovirus
    C. Phenytoin
    D. Warfarin

4.62. Pathogenic variants in which gene may contribute to Alzheimer disease suscepti-bility, but, unlike the others, does NOT cause or appear to primarily contribute to early-onset familial Alzheimer disease?
    A. *APOE*
    B. *APP*
    C. *PSEN1*
    D. *PSEN2*

4.63. Carrier status related to which of the conditions below is more common in people of Ashkenazi Jewish ancestry?
    A. Cystic fibrosis
    B. Gaucher disease
    C. Tay-Sachs disease
    D. All of the above

4.64. Genetic changes in what gene are most strongly associated with the risk of a type of chronic kidney disease?
    A. *APOE*
    B. *APOL1*
    C. *HTT*
    D. *OR6A2*

4.65. Pathogenic variants in what two genes cause Kabuki syndrome?
    A. *COL11A1* and *COL11A2*
    B. *EYA1* and *SIX1*
    C. *KMT2D* and *KDM6A*
    D. *SHH* and *ZIC2*

4.66. Which of the following is true regarding noninvasive prenatal screening (NIPS)?
    A. Can screen for aneuploidies and other conditions
    B. Is least accurate for trisomy 21
    C. Requires amniocentesis
    D. Requires a paternal blood sample

4.67. The American College of Medical Genetics and Genomics (ACMG) recommends reporting secondary findings in certain genes. This list continues to evolve; INITIALLY, findings in approximately how many genes were recommended for return in individuals undergoing clinical exome or genome sequencing?
    A. 0–5
    B. 50–100
    C. 500–1000
    D. 10 000–200 000

4.68. The presence of succinylacetone on newborn screening is indicative of what condition?
    A. Hypothyroidism
    B. Maple syrup urine disease
    C. Severe combined immunodeficiency
    D. Tyrosinemia type I

4.69. Pathogenic variants in which group of genes can result in dermatologic conditions such as epidermolysis bullosa, pachyonychia congenita, and forms of ichthyosis?
A. Hedgehog
B. Homeobox
C. Keratin
D. Myosin

4.70. A cohort of patients have been described to be affected with findings such as ectodermal dysplasia, cleft lip/palate, and ectrodactyly. What gene would most likely be involved to explain the findings in this cohort?
A. *FLNA*
B. *LMNA*
C. *TP53*
D. *TP63*

4.71. A patient has clinical features strongly compatible with a specific microdeletion syndrome (involving a deletion of ~2.5 Mb). Which test would be LEAST likely to confirm the genetic diagnosis?
A. FISH
B. Karyotype
C. Microarray
D. Exome (with reliable CNV calling)

4.72. Which of the following genes is involved in conditions that include hereditary disposition to hyperparathyroidism and increased risk of certain types of cancer?
A. *BRCA1*
B. *BRCA2*
C. *CDC73*
D. *CDH1*

4.73. A patient with cancer undergoes tumor-based genetic testing. A genetic change is identified in the tumor sample; germline genetic testing does not identify this genetic change. What is the best way to describe this variant?
A. Artifactual
B. Constitutional
C. Germline
D. Somatic

4.74. Which pair of conditions is allelic (caused by genetic changes in the same gene)?
A. Becker muscular dystrophy and Duchenne muscular dystrophy
B. Emery-Dreifuss muscular dystrophy and Nemaline myopathy
C. Fascioscapulohumeral muscular dystrophy and Ullrich congenital muscular dystrophy
D. Rigid spine muscular dystrophy and Oculopharyngeal muscular dystrophy

4.75. Variants in the gene *HOXB13* is associated with hereditary predisposition to what condition?
A. Cardiomyopathy
B. Peripheral neuropathy
C. Prostate cancer
D. Sarcoidosis

4.76. Pathogenic variants in which gene cause Acute intermittent porphyria?
A. *HBB*
B. *HMBS*
C. *HOXB1*
D. *HTT*

4.77. Arginenemia, Maple syrup urine disease, Phenylketonuria, and Tyrosinemia all belong to what category of inborn error of metabolism?
A. Amino acidemia
B. Fatty acid oxidation disorder
C. Lysosomal storage disorder
D. Urea cycle disorder

4.78. A patient undergoes clinical genome sequencing. Through secondary analysis, a pathogenic variant is found in a gene involving an increased risk of cancer. In which of the following genes was this variant most likely found?

A. *APOB*

B. *BMPR1A*

C. *COL3A1*

D. *RYR1*

4.79. A study involves conducting whole-genome sequencing in a cohort of many thousands of previously untested patients with different, suspected Mendelian genetic conditions. For those for whom answers are found, most of the causative pathogenic variants are likely to be in which portion of the genome?

A. Exons

B. Introns

C. Telomeres

D. UTR

4.80. Variants in which of the following genes is NOT considered to be associated with monogenic causes of Parkinson disease?

A. *GBA*

B. *HTRA1*

C. *LRRK2*

D. *PRKN*

4.81. Which of the following are encoded by the human histocompatibility complex genes? That is, which are encoded by the human version of the major histocompatibility complex (MHC) gene group?

A. Acylcarnitine

B. Homeobox

C. Human leukocyte antigen

D. Tumor necrosis factor

4.82. Pathogenic variants in which gene are a relatively frequent cause of Hereditary spherocytosis?

A. *ANK1*

B. *ENG*

C. *HBB*

D. *VWF*

4.83. Which type of molar pregnancy contains only genetic material from the father, and involves a higher risk of progression to choriocarcinoma?

A. Asymptomatic

B. Complete

C. Partial

D. Recurrent

4.84. An adult with cancer is noted to have trichilemmomas and papillomatous papules. What gene is most likely to be involved?

A. *BRCA1*

B. *PTEN*

C. *TP53*

D. *VHL*

4.85. A child with signs of a neurological condition has been found to have galactocerebrosidase deficiency. What condition is caused by deficiency of this enzyme?

A. Gaucher disease

B. Hunter syndrome

C. Krabbe disease

D. Sly syndrome

4.86. Which genes/proteins are involved in many skeletal dysplasias (as well as other disorders)?

A. Ankyrin

B. Collagen

C. Sodium channel

D. Spectrin

4.87. Which of the following refers to a term for a variant of galactosemia, which involves partial galactose-1-phosphate uridylyltransferase deficiency?

A. Delta F508

B. Duarte

C. Hemoglobin Bart's

D. Thalassemia major

4.88. Which of the following conditions has the highest de novo rate (that is, has individuals who are most likely to have the condition due to a de novo pathogenic variant versus inheriting the causative pathogenic variant from an affected parent)?
A. Achondroplasia
B. Marfan syndrome
C. Neurofibromatosis type 1
D. Tuberous sclerosis complex

4.89. Which category of genetic condition can be caused by pathogenic variants in genes including *BRAF, KRAS, NF1, PTPN11, RAF1, RIT1, SOS1,* and *SPRED1* (as well as other genes)?
A. Autoinflammatory
B. Organic acidemia
C. Primary immunodeficiency
D. RASopathy

4.90. A patient has clinical features involved in 22q11.2 deletion syndrome but microarray is normal. Which gene might be involved?
A. *ELN*
B. *PAFAH1B1*
C. *RAI1*
D. *TBX1*

4.91. Which of the following conditions is due to somatic (versus germline/constitutional) pathogenic variants?
A. Li-Fraumeni syndrome
B. Fanconi anemia
C. Proteus syndrome
D. Zellweger syndrome

4.92. On examination, a patient is noted to have "coarse" facial features. Based on this finding, which type of testing would most likely be indicated to try to identify the cause of the person's condition?
A. Chromosomal breakage studies
B. FISH for 22q11.2
C. *FMR1* repeat analysis
D. Urine glycosaminoglycans

4.93. A patient has features consistent with Turner syndrome. Assuming this is the correct diagnosis, what result would be expected on routine cytogenomic studies (with the caveat that mosaic results are not uncommon)?
A. 45,X
B. 45,XO
C. 46,XX
D. 47,XXX

4.94. A person undergoes genetic testing because of a strong family history of papillary renal cell carcinoma. Which of the following genes would most likely be indicated for inclusion in a genetic testing panel for this patient?
A. *ANKRD26*
B. *MET*
C. *RET*
D. *STK11*

4.95. An infant boy has a scaly skin rash. Assuming a genetic diagnosis, deficiency of what enzyme might be suspected?
A. Aldolase B
B. Arginase
C. Mevalonate kinase
D. Steroid sulfatase

Answers

4.1. C	4.4. C	4.7. B	4.10. B
4.2. C	4.5. C	4.8. C	4.11. A
4.3. B	4.6. A	4.9. C	4.12. B

4.13.	C	4.34.	C	4.55.	C	4.76.	B
4.14.	B	4.35.	B	4.56.	C	4.77.	A
4.15.	D	4.36.	C	4.57.	D	4.78.	B
4.16.	B	4.37.	A	4.58.	A	4.79.	A
4.17.	D	4.38.	A	4.59.	D	4.80.	B
4.18.	C	4.39.	D	4.60.	B	4.81.	C
4.19.	D	4.40.	A	4.61.	D	4.82.	A
4.20.	B	4.41.	A	4.62.	A	4.83.	B
4.21.	C	4.42.	B	4.63.	D	4.84.	B
4.22.	D	4.43.	C	4.64.	B	4.85.	C
4.23.	D	4.44.	C	4.65.	C	4.86.	B
4.24.	A	4.45.	A	4.66.	A	4.87.	B
4.25.	C	4.46.	B	4.67.	B	4.88.	A
4.26.	C	4.47.	C	4.68.	D	4.89.	D
4.27.	D	4.48.	A	4.69.	C	4.90.	D
4.28.	B	4.49.	A	4.70.	D	4.91.	C
4.29.	D	4.50.	B	4.71.	B	4.92.	D
4.30.	A	4.51.	C	4.72.	C	4.93.	A
4.31.	B	4.52.	C	4.73.	D	4.94.	B
4.32.	D	4.53.	A	4.74.	A	4.95.	D
4.33.	A	4.54.	C	4.75.	C		

Commentary

4.1. *CDH1*

Up to ~3% of gastric cancer worldwide has been attributed to inherited cancer predisposition syndromes. Heterozygous pathogenic variants in the gene *CDH1* result in increased risk for Hereditary diffuse gastric cancer. However, most people who meet clinical criteria for Hereditary diffuse gastric cancer syndrome do not have germline pathogenic variants identified in *CDH1*. *CDH1* pathogenic variants resulting in Hereditary diffuse gastric cancer are usually inherited in an autosomal dominant fashion, though de novo pathogenic variants have also been reported. Most gastric cancer in *CDH1*-positive individuals occurs by age 40; the risk by 80 years of age has been estimated to be up to ~70% in men and ~56% in women. Women are also at increased risk of lobular breast cancer (~42% risk by 80 years of age). In addition to *CDH1*, pathogenic variants in other genes can also confer increased risk of gastric cancer.

Reference(s): Kaurah and Huntsman [1]; van der Post et al. [2]; Petrovchich and Ford [3].

4.2. Premutation allele

Fragile X syndrome (FXS) is the most common form of inherited intellectual disability. FXS is caused by an increased number of CGG trinucleotide repeats in the *FMR1* gene, which is located on the X chromosome (a very small fraction of patients can have other types of genetic changes affecting the gene). Both males and females with "full mutation" alleles can have FXS, though females are typically more mildly and less frequently affected. *FMR1* alleles are classified by the number of trinucleotide repeats:

Normal allele: ~5–44 repeats
Intermediate allele: ~45–54 repeats
Premutation allele: ~55–200 repeats
Full mutation allele: >200 repeats

A premutation allele (using standard but perhaps semantically questionable terminology) may expand to a full mutation allele when passed down from a mother to a child. Similarly, an intermediate allele may expand to a premutation allele when passed down from a mother to a child. In addition to the risk of having a child with FXS, a premutation allele can cause Fragile X tremor ataxia syndrome (FXTAS), which includes late-onset cerebellar ataxia and tremor, or FMR1-related primary ovarian insufficiency.

Reference(s): Bagni et al. [4]; Hunter et al. [5].

4.3. Chronic granulomatous disease

Chronic granulomatous disease (CGD) involves severe recurrent bacterial and fungal infections and inflammatory dysregulation, and results in granuloma formation and other inflammatory conditions such as colitis, which may be the only or initial finding. CGD is caused by pathogenic variants affecting the genes encoding subunits of phagocyte NADPH oxidase. The inheritance is autosomal recessive or X-linked. In addition to molecular testing, CGD may be diagnosed by testing that measures neutrophil superoxide production by the NADPH oxidase complex, including the dihydrorhodamine (DHR) test, which is used more frequently than the older nitroblue tetrazolium (NBT) test.

Reference(s): Leiding and Holland [6]; Arnold and Heimall [7].

4.4. Buccal swab or skin biopsy

Pallister-Killian syndrome, sometimes called Pallister-Killian mosaic syndrome, is caused by mosaic tetrasomy of chromosome 12p (typically involving an additional isochromosome 12). Manifestations are variable, but can include neurocognitive impairment, seizures, and distinctive features on physical examination, as well as other findings. Blood-based chromosomal testing will not typically detect the causative cytogenomic anomalies, but testing via buccal swab (which is easier to conduct, but involves some limitations) or skin biopsy can identify the cytogenomic cause.

Reference(s): Manasse et al. [8]; Karaman et al. [9]; Bertini et al. [10].

4.5. *BRCA2*

Germline pathogenic variants in a number of genes have been implicated as increasing the risk of prostate cancer. Among these, pathogenic variants in *BRCA2* have been most commonly implicated. *BRCA2* is also involved in other cancer types in both men and women. In terms of treatment implications, and in addition to other benefits, knowledge of germline or somatic pathogenic variants in DNA repair genes (such as *BRCA2*) in patients with prostate cancer may yield therapeutic possibilities, such as with poly-ADP ribose polymerase (PARP) inhibitors.

Reference(s): Leongamornlert et al. [11]; Mateo et al. [12]; Pritchard et al. [13]; Giri et al. [14].

4.6. Karyotype

Though increasingly replaced by newer molecular technologies in a variety of clinical contexts, the karyotype can be a useful, efficient, and available assay to visualize the chromosomes in certain scenarios. Karyotype can be used to detect balanced translocations; some other technologies, such as the other choices mentioned will not typically be able to detect these translocations, either because they are too limited in scope in terms of the genetic/genomic information evaluated, or because they do not provide adequate information about the physical arrangement or location of genetic/genomic material.

Reference(s): Wilch and Morton [15]; Nussbaum et al. [16].

4.7. PI*Z

Alpha-1 antitrypsin deficiency (AATD) involves increased risk for adult lung disease (chronic obstructive pulmonary disease) and child or adult liver disease. Other features, such as panniculitis, may also occur. Environmental factors like smoking can exacerbate the condition. AATD is an autosomal recessive condition caused by pathogenic variants in the gene *SERPINA1*. The most common pathogenic allele, using one nomenclature, is termed PI*Z (but can also go by other terms, such as PiZ or Z). This allele is more common in individuals of northern European ancestry. AATD occurs in about 1 in 5000–7000 North Americans but 1 in 1500–3000 Scandinavians. The most common unaffected allele is termed PI*M. "PI" refers to Protease Inhibitor, another name for the gene. In addition to these two alleles, many others have been described.

Reference(s): Stoller and Aboussouan [17]; Greene et al. [18]; Stoller et al. [19].

4.8. *PTPN11*

Noonan syndrome, like many genetic conditions, can be caused by pathogenic variants in multiple different genes – this phenomenon is termed genetic heterogeneity. Among patients with Noonan syndrome, pathogenic variants in the gene *PTPN11* are the most frequently identified (in about 50% of individuals). Pathogenic variants in other genes can also cause the condition, and some genotype–phenotype correlations have been suggested. Variants in these genes may also be related to other conditions.

Reference(s): Allanson and Roberts [20]; Liao and Mehta [21].

4.9. Prader-Willi syndrome

Many genetic conditions can be molecularly diagnosed via modalities such as exome or genome sequencing. These approaches can be especially useful for heterogeneous disorders and other conditions that may be difficult to recognize. Lab-based and bioinformatic improvements are enabling the detection of a broader range of potential disease-related variants. Some conditions, however, may require or be best detected by a specific, separate assay. One example of such a condition is Prader-Willi syndrome (PWS). PWS is due to changes affecting a region of chromosome 15q11.2–q13. These changes can include paternal deletion, maternal uniparental disomy (UPD), or an imprinting defect affecting this region. When PWS is suspected, methylation testing of the affected region may be performed.

Reference(s): Biesecker and Green [22]; Driscoll et al. [23].

4.10. *SCN1A*

Dravet syndrome is defined as a rare genetic epileptic encephalopathy in an otherwise healthy infant, with onset during the first year of life. Approximately 80% of patients with diagnosed Dravet syndrome have a heterozygous pathogenic variant in *SCN1A*, which usually occurs de novo. Infants with Dravet syndrome may have a variety of different seizure types, which may be frequent and treatment-refractory. Variants in other genes can also cause Dravet syndrome. Pathogenic variants in *SCN1A* can also cause other seizure-related conditions, including milder forms of epilepsy.

Reference(s): Helbig and Tayoun [24]; Miller and Sotero de Menezes [25]; Wheless et al. [26].

4.11. Alkaptonuria

In the United States, newborn screening (NBS) has been established on a state-by-state basis with a goal of efficiently and cost-effectively identifying infants who have conditions for which early treatment is available and necessary to ameliorate disease. The Recommended Uniform Screening Panel (RUSP) is a list of disorders that the Secretary of the Department of Health and Human Services (HHS) recommends for inclusion. Disorders are chosen based on evidence that supports potential screening benefits, state abilities, and treatment availability. HHS recommends that every infant undergo NBS for all RUSP conditions. Each state's public health department decides which conditions are included in its NBS program. Most states screen for the majority of RUSP-recommended conditions, and some states screen for additional disorders not on the RUSP. Alkaptonuria, an autosomal recessive biochemical condition that can affect the joints and other organ systems, is not currently part of NBS conditions.

Reference(s): American College of Medical Genetics and Genomics ACT Sheets and Confirmatory Algorithms [27]; US Department of Health and Human Services, Advisory Committee on Heritable Disorders in Newborns and Children [28].

4.12. *TP53*

Heterozygous pathogenic variants in the gene *TP53* cause Li-Fraumeni syndrome. A variety of neoplasms may affect patients, and these may occur in childhood or adulthood. Characteristic neoplasms include adrenocortical carcinoma, brain tumors, leukemia, osteosarcoma, premenopausal breast cancer, and soft tissue sarcoma. Patients are frequently affected with early-onset cancer and multiple primary tumors. Most variants are inherited in an autosomal dominant manner, but ~7–20% of pathogenic variants are estimated to occur de novo. In addition to germline pathogenic variants related to Li-Fraumeni syndrome, somatic pathogenic variants in *TP53* can play an important role in the development and progression of cancer.

Reference(s): McBride et al. [29]; Schneider et al. [30].

4.13. Genetic prion disorders

Familial Creutzfeldt-Jakob disease, Gerstmann-Sträussler-Scheinker (GSS) syndrome, and Fatal familial insomnia are all considered genetic prion disorders.

The manifestations may vary between conditions and among patients, but can include ataxia, cognitive difficulties, and myoclonus. Pathogenic variants in the *PRNP* gene can cause these conditions. Prion diseases can also be due to acquired causes, through infectious mechanisms.

Reference(s): Ironside et al. [31]; Tee et al. [32]; Zerr and Schmitz [33].

4.14. *GNAQ*

Both "port-wine stains," which are cutaneous vascular malformations, and Sturge-Weber syndrome (SWS) can be due to somatic pathogenic variants in the *GNAQ* gene. SWS is a sporadic condition that also involves seizures, glaucoma, and intracranial vascular anomalies (leptomeningeal angiomatosis), especially involving the occipital and posterior parietal lobes. Infants born with a facial port-wine stain have been reported as having an ~6% chance of having SWS; when the port-wine stain is located in the distribution of the ophthalmic branch of the trigeminal nerve, this risk has been estimated to be ~25%. Of note, SWS does not frequently involve dermatologic lesions in non-facial areas. The molecular etiologies of these conditions were initially found by sequencing affected compared to unaffected tissue; a single genetic change in the *GNAQ* gene (c.548G>A, resulting in p.Arg183Gln) was found to be causative.

Reference(s): Hall et al. [34]; Ch'ng and Tan [35]; Piram et al. [36]; Shirley et al. [37].

4.15. Sotos

Sotos syndrome can be caused by heterozygous microdeletions of chromosome 5q35 or pathogenic variants in the gene *NSD1*, which is located on 5q35. Deletions have been described as more common in individuals of Japanese ancestry. The condition typically includes a distinctive craniofacial appearance, overgrowth, and intellectual disability. It has been suggested that patients with microdeletions may have less overgrowth but more severe learning disability than patients with *NSD1* pathogenic variants. The differential diagnosis can include other overgrowth conditions, such as Beckwith-Wiedemann, Simpson-Golabi-Behmel, and Weaver-Smith syndromes.

Reference(s): Foster et al. [38]; Tatton-Brown et al. [39]; Jones et al. [40].

4.16. C9ORF72

Amyotrophic lateral sclerosis (ALS) is the most common adult-onset motor neuron disease. ALS is characterized by upper and/or lower motor neuron dysfunction, which leads to progressive muscle weakness and respiratory insufficiency. Frontotemporal lobar degeneration (FTLD) is the second most common cause of dementia in adults under 65 years of age. FTLD manifests as changes in behavior, executive dysfunction, and language impairment. An increased number of hexanucleotide repeats in *C9ORF72* can cause ALS and/or FTLD. Alleles with disease-causing increased repeats can be inherited in an autosomal dominant manner or can occur de novo. *C9ORF72*-related disease manifestations may initially include only ALS or FTLD, but many affected individuals will present with features of both disorders as well as features of Parkinsonism. The age of onset typically ranges from about 30 to 70 years of age.

Reference(s): Haeusler et al. [41]; Gijselinck et al. [42].

Chapter 4

4.17. Severe combined immunodeficiency

Newborn screening (NBS) for certain types of immunodeficiencies is performed using T-cell receptor excision circle (TREC) assays. The TREC assays are performed on dried blood spots (DBS) collected shortly after birth. TRECs are a biomarker of T-cell generation. Low TREC concentrations reflect T-cell lymphopenia (TCL). Immunodeficiencies were incorporated into NBS programs in 2010 after Severe combined immunodeficiency (SCID) was added to the core conditions listed in the Recommended Uniform Screening Panel (RUSP). SCID is one type of primary immunodeficiency. SCID includes severe TCL, which leads to recurrent and severe infections, failure to thrive, and death within the first year if untreated. Less than 20% of patients with SCID are diagnosed based on family history; survival is improved when SCID is diagnosed and treated early and before the onset of infection, such as through NBS.

References: Pai et al. [43]; Kwan and Puck [44].

4.18. *MUTYH*

Biallelic germline pathogenic variants in the gene *MUTYH* result in *MUTYH*-associated polyposis (MAP). MAP includes greatly increased colorectal cancer risk, as well as additional gastrointestinal neoplasms such as duodenal adenomas and hyperplastic/serrated adenomas. Heterozygous pathogenic variants in *MLH1*, *MSH2*, *MSH6*, and *PMS2*, and heterozygous deletions in *EPCAM* cause Lynch syndrome. Biallelic pathogenic variants in these genes (though not *EPCAM*) cause Constitutional mismatch repair deficiency syndrome, a rare childhood cancer predisposition syndrome that involves brain/central nervous system tumors, colorectal cancer and intestinal polyps, hematologic malignancies, and other malignancies.

Reference(s): Sampson et al. [45]; Wimmer and Kratz [46]; Nielsen et al. [47].

4.19. Hemoglobin S

Sickle cell disease (SCD) is an autosomal recessive condition that can be caused by a hemoglobin S allele (pathogenic variant in the *HBB* gene, resulting in p.Glu6Val) in conjunction with another pathogenic variant affecting *HBB*, including a hemoglobin S allele, a hemoglobin C allele, a β+-thalassemia or β°-thalassemia allele, or hemoglobin D, O, E, or other beta globin chain variant allele. SCD involves chronic hemolytic anemia and intermittent vaso-occlusive events that can affect multiple organ systems.

Reference(s): Piel et al. [48]; Bender [49].

4.20. *RAI1*

Smith-Magenis syndrome (SMS), which involves intellectual disability, behavioral differences, and distinct craniofacial and skeletal findings, is caused by heterozygous deletion of chromosome 17p11.2. Heterozygous pathogenic variants in the gene *RAI1*, which is located in the SMS chromosomal region, can also cause the condition.

Reference(s): Slager et al. [50]; Smith et al. [51].

4.21. *MECP2*

Pathogenic variants in the X-linked gene *MECP2* can result in a spectrum of conditions in females, including classic Rett syndrome, variant Rett syndrome, and mild learning disabilities. Stages of disease in patients with classic Rett syndrome include apparently normal cognitive development for the first approximately 6–18 months of life; a short period of developmental stagnation; a period of rapid developmental regression; long-term stability. In males, pathogenic variants in this gene are typically lethal, though severe neonatal encephalopathy with other neurocognitive effects has been described.

Reference(s): Neul et al. [52]; Leonard et al. [53]; Kaur et al. [54].

4.22. Zinc

Multiple genetic disorders are due to abnormalities related to the metabolism of different metals, including copper, iron, and zinc. Of these, Acrodermatitis enteropathica, Birk-Landau-Perez syndrome, and Spondylocheirodysplastic Ehlers-Danlos syndrome, as well as Transient neonatal zinc deficiency, involve abnormal zinc metabolism.

Reference(s): Ferreira and Gahl [55].

4.23. *STK11*

Peutz-Jeghers syndrome (PJS) is an autosomal dominant condition due to pathogenic variants in the gene *STK11*. Clinical features include mucocutaneous pigmentation, gastrointestinal polyposis (most frequently small bowel, but also affecting other GI and non-GI areas), and cancer predisposition, including epithelial cancers, sex cord tumors with annular tubules (SCTAT), cervical adenoma malignum, and Sertoli cell tumors of the testes. The mucocutaneous pigmentation can include dark pigmented macules around the mouth (and buccal mucosa), eyes, and nostrils, in the perianal area, and hyperpigmented areas on the fingers.

Reference(s): Beggs et al. [56]; McGarrity et al. [57].

4.24. Adrenoleukodystrophy

X-linked adrenoleukodystrophy (X-ALD) is caused by pathogenic variants in *ABCD1*. Affected males may demonstrate one of three main clinical conditions: a childhood cerebral form, adrenomyeloneuropathy, or a form presenting initially with Addison disease and typically including neurologic manifestations by middle age. Approximately one-quarter of females with pathogenic variants demonstrate some manifestations in adulthood. Diagnosis relies on characteristic clinical and laboratory-based testing. Early diagnosis is important in order to allow optimal disease management.

Reference(s): Shapiro et al. [58]; Raymond et al. [59].

4.25. *L1CAM*

Pathogenic variants in the X-linked gene *L1CAM* can cause a number of neurologic conditions. Congenital hydrocephalus due to aqueductal stenosis may be observed as an isolated finding, but is frequently associated with other features, including hypoplastic or flexed, adducted thumbs, varying degrees of intellectual disability, and spastic paraplegia. Pathogenic variants can also cause other conditions with overlapping features. There can be significant phenotypic variability, including within families. About 5% of women with *L1CAM* pathogenic variants exhibit clinical manifestations. Prenatally, genetic testing of *L1CAM* may be considered in male fetuses with hydrocephalus, especially when hypoplastic or adducted thumbs are noted and/or there is a suggestive family history, as well as for female fetuses with hydrocephalus due to aqueductal stenosis.

Reference(s): Tully and Dobyns [60]; Stumpel and Vos [61].

4.26. p.Cys282Tyr

Hereditary hemochromatosis is a genetic iron overload disorder. The condition is caused by excess iron absorption by the gastrointestinal mucosa. The clinical spectrum is wide, ranging from clinically and biochemically asymptomatic to symptomatic individuals. Clinical signs and symptoms, when present, can be initially nonspecific, but involve end-organ damage due to iron overload. This damage can affect multiple organs, including the liver as well as the heart, joints, pancreas, skin, and testes. Biochemical signs include elevated transferrin-iron saturation and serum ferritin concentration. Biallelic pathogenic variants in the *HFE* gene can cause Hereditary hemochromatosis, though there are other genetic causes. Among common variants in the *HFE* gene, p.Cys282Tyr has been identified in ~10% of non-Hispanic white individuals; ~25% of non-Hispanic white individuals carry p.His63Asp, though homozygosity for the latter variant is not believed to independently cause disease.

Reference(s): Adams [62]; Barton and Edwards [63]; Nussbaum et al. [16].

4.27. All of the above

In genetics, variant classification is a dynamic process. That is, re-evaluating variants is an intrinsic part of the genetic testing/evaluation process. As part of this process, variants may be reclassified in terms of their potential pathogenicity. Variants may be reclassified for multiple possible reasons, including new functional, population, and segregation data.

Reference(s): Richards et al. [64]; Mersch et al. [65]; Deignan et al. [66]; Harrison and Rehm [67].

4.28. *DICER1*

DICER1 pathogenic variants cause a condition that includes elevated risk for pleuropulmonary blastoma (PPB) as well as other neoplasms, including (in alphabetical order) Botryoid-type embryonal rhabdomyosarcoma, ciliary body medulloepithelioma, cystic nephroma, nasal chondromesenchymal hamartoma, nodular thyroid hyperplasia, ovarian sex-cord stromal tumors, pineoblastoma, pituitary blastoma, and others. PPBs can occur in early childhood, and often present with respiratory symptoms. Overall, most tumors occur before the age of 40 years.

Reference(s): Schultz et al. [68]; Schultz et al. [69].

4.29. Glucocerebrosidase

Gaucher disease (GD) is an autosomal recessive lysosomal storage disorder caused by pathogenic variants in *GBA*, causing deficient glucocerebrosidase (also called glucosylceramidase as well as by other terms) enzyme activity. The condition has a very broad range of manifestations, ranging from perinatal lethal to asymptomatic. GD can be diagnosed enzymatically, with the diagnosis confirmed by molecular testing. Management may involve enzyme replacement therapy (ERT) or substrate reduction therapy (SRT), as well as symptomatic treatment (e.g. splenectomy) and supportive care.

Reference(s): Mistry et al. [70]; Pastores and Hughes [71].

4.30. *IKBKG*

Incontinentia pigmenti (IP) is an X-linked dominant condition caused by pathogenic variants in the gene *IKBKG* (also called *NEMO*). The condition affects multiple organ systems. Skin findings, which follow the lines of Blaschko, evolve through multiple stages, including erythema and blistering (birth to ~24 months); wart-like rash, mainly on the limbs (first weeks of life to ~24 months); hyperpigmented streaks and whorls (~4 months to ~16 years); atrophic/hypopigmented linear streaks (adolescence through adulthood). In addition to skin findings, other clinical manifestations can include alopecia, dental anomalies (hypodontia and dysplastic teeth), nail dystrophy, retinal neovascularization and subsequent detachment, and neurocognitive dysfunction. There are also several allelic conditions caused by pathogenic variants in the same gene. In males, IP is embryonic lethal.

Reference(s): Scheuerle and Urisini [72]; Jones et al. [40].

4.31. Aicardi-Goutières syndrome

Newborn screening uses a combination of methods to detect selected, potentially treatable conditions. Screening for X-linked adrenoleukodystrophy (X-ALD) involves assessing for the presence of abnormal levels of C26 : 0 lysophosphatidylcholine. A number of patients with Aicardi-Goutières syndrome (AGS) have been identified through newborn screening for X-ALD. It is characterized by central nervous system calcifications, leukodystrophy, and neurocognitive impairment, and can be caused by pathogenic variants in multiple genes. One hint about the possibility of AGS in patients who screen positive for X-ALD involves the presence of early-onset neurological manifestations.

Reference(s): Rice et al. [73]; Armangue et al. [74]; Lee et al. [75]; Tise et al. [76].

4.32. *PMS2*

Lynch syndrome, which can be caused by pathogenic variants in several genes involved in DNA mismatch repair, involves an increased risk of colorectal, endometrial, and other types of cancer. In people with suspected Lynch syndrome, genetic testing for germline variants is often conducted by examining all of the Lynch syndrome genes at once, including as part of a larger panel of cancer-related genes. Of the Lynch syndrome genes, *PMS2* testing and interpretation is complicated by the presence of several large pseudogenes. When certain genetic variants are identified, it is clinically important to differentiate whether they occur in *PMS2* or in a pseudogene.

Reference(s): Hegde et al. [77]; Idos and Valle [78].

4.33. African

Cardiac amyloidosis, which typically manifests as progressive cardiomyopathy, can be caused by heterozygous pathogenic variants in the *TTR* gene. It is estimated that ~3–4% of African-Americans harbor the p.Val122Ile variant in *TTR*. Cardiac amyloidosis is one phenotype in the overall TTR-related condition known as Familial transthyretin amyloidosis, which also includes Familial amyloid polyneuropathy, Leptomeningeal amyloidosis, and Familial oculoleptomeningeal amyloidosis (FOLMA).

Reference(s): Ruberg and Berk [79]; Sekijima [80].

Chapter 4

4.34. *SPRED1*

Legius syndrome is a RASopathy caused by heterozygous pathogenic variants in the gene *SPRED1*. The condition involves the presence of multiple café au lait macules but without neurofibromas or other tumor manifestations of Neurofibromatosis type 1; other common findings include developmental delay and learning disabilities, attention deficit hyperactivity disorder, lipomas, macrocephaly, and intertriginous freckling.

Reference(s): Rauen [81]; Legius and Stevenson [82].

4.35. Bloom syndrome

Bloom syndrome is an autosomal recessive condition caused by biallelic pathogenic variants in the gene *BLM* (*RECQL3*). Clinical features include prenatal and postnatal growth deficiency, decreased subcutaneous fat, distinctive craniofacial features, feeding problems early in life, mild immunodeficiency (low immunoglobulins and increased risk of otitis media and pneumonia), photosensitivity with red skin lesions on the nose and cheek, male infertility, early menopause, learning difficulties and/or intellectual disability in some individuals, and an increased risk of multiple cancer types at a younger age than in the general population. Molecular testing can be used for diagnosis; cytogenetic studies that show increased sister chromatid exchange may also be helpful.

Reference(s): Flanagan and Cunniff [83].

4.36. *CDKN2A*

About 2% of people develop melanoma in their lifetime. Malignant melanoma (MM) usually occurs in people with no family history, but about 10% of those with MM have at least one first- or second-degree relative with a history of MM. While germline pathogenic variants in multiple genes can cause or contribute to MM, evidence shows that about 20–40% (with the reported range depending on study characteristics such as inclusion criteria) of familial MM is thought to be due to pathogenic germline variants in the gene *CDKN2A*. Pathogenic variants in genes related to MM can also cause or contribute to the development of other cancer types. Somatic pathogenic variants in other genes are also important biomarkers.

Reference(s): NCI Surveillance Research Program [84]; Leachman et al. [85].

4.37. Droplet digital PCR

The clinical relevance of mosaic variants is becoming increasingly appreciated, including the fact that these variants can impact many different genes and clinical conditions. There are different ways to assess mosaicism. Droplet digital polymerase chain reaction (ddPCR) enables the quantification of specifically targeted genetic variants via counting the proportion of the targeted nucleic acid molecules present. ddPCR can be used to precisely detect a variety of types of genetic changes, including those present at levels too low for other methods to reliably detect. This method is used increasingly in research contexts and may also be available in some clinical scenarios.

Reference(s): Vogelstein et al. [86]; Lindy et al. [87]; Zhou et al. [88]; Beck et al. [89].

4.38. *DMPK*

Myotonic dystrophy type 1 (DM1) results from expansion of a CTG trinucleotide repeat in the noncoding region of the *DMPK* gene. The condition affects multiple organ systems, including skeletal and smooth muscle as well as the heart, eye, and central nervous system. Clinical manifestations can have a wide range, but have been categorized into three types: congenital, classic, and mild disease. Myotonic dystrophy type 2 (DM2) is a clinically overlapping condition caused by expansion of a CCTG repeat in the *CNBP* gene.

Reference(s): Udd and Krahe [90]; Bird [91].

4.39. Sarcomere

Hypertrophic cardiomyopathy (HCM) occurs in about 1 in 500 individuals. The onset of HCM may range from neonatal to adult, and the condition may have a highly variable course, ranging from asymptompatically affected individuals to a lethal condition that can manifest with sudden cardiac death. Multiple causative genes have been identified, and genetic forms may follow autosomal dominant, autosomal recessive, or X-linked inheritance patterns. In the genetic forms of HCM, pathogenic variants cause disease by their effects on the sarcomere, which is a unit of striated muscle. That is, pathogenic variants in genes that encode for sarcomere components can cause HCM.

Reference(s): Ingles et al. [92]; Cirini and Ho [93].

4.40. *EXT1, EXT2*

Hereditary multiple osteochondromas (HMO) (sometimes referred to as hereditary multiple exostoses) involves the presence of multiple osteochondromas, which are benign bone tumors growing from the long bone metaphyses. These osteochondromas can cause sequelae such as reduced skeletal growth and skeletal deformity, reduced stature, osteoarthrosis, and peripheral nerve compression. Osteochondromas may undergo malignant degeneration, though the lifetime risk is ~1%. The condition can be caused by heterozygous pathogenic variants affecting the *EXT1* or *EXT2* genes; these variants can include large deletions that may affect other genes, such as in Langer-Giedion syndrome, a separate condition.

Reference(s): Wuyts et al. [94]; Jones et al. [40].

4.41. GWAS

A genome-wide association study (GWAS) is a method for identifying genetic variants that may be associated with a certain condition. In a GWAS, in general, genetic variants in people with the condition are compared to genetic variants in people without the condition to see which variants may be statistically significantly over- or under-represented in each group. The particular platform used for genetic testing may vary depending on the study, but many GWAS traditionally used genome-wide single-nucleotide polymorphism arrays. Many thousands of GWAS have been conducted and published since the first such studies were described.

Reference(s): Klein et al. [95]; Tam et al. [96].

4.42. *GJB2*

There are many genetic (as well as nongenetic) causes of hearing loss. In developed countries, about 80% of congenital hearing loss is estimated to be due to genetic causes. Genetic causes may be nonsyndromic or syndromic, and inheritance may be autosomal dominant, autosomal recessive, X-linked, or mitochondrial. The type and severity of hearing loss also varies according to the underlying cause. It has been estimated that around half of severe-to-profound autosomal recessive nonsyndromic hearing loss results from biallelic pathogenic variants (mutations) in the gene *GJB2*, which encodes connexin 26.

Reference(s): Sloan-Heggen et al. [97]; Shearer et al. [98].

4.43. Exon 8 (old literature: exon 7) loss

Spinal Muscular Atrophy (SMA) involves muscle weakness and atrophy due to progressive degeneration and loss of the anterior horn cells in the spinal cord and brain stem nuclei. SMA can be caused by biallelic pathogenic variants (mutations) in the *SMN1* gene. Loss of exon 8 (referred to as exon 7 in older literature) is the most common such pathogenic variant. Disease severity is modified by the dosage (copy number) of *SMN2*. Pathogenic variants in other genes can also cause different types of SMA and similar conditions.

Reference(s): Prior and Finanger [99].

4.44. *LMNA*

Hutchinson-Gilford progeria syndrome (HGPS) is caused by heterozygous pathogenic variants in the *LMNA* gene. The condition resembles accelerated/premature aging, and includes early failure to thrive, a characteristic facial appearance, alopecia, loss of subcutaneous fat, joint contractures, bone, and nail changes, as well as hearing loss and dental anomalies. While "classic" HGPS is diagnosed through a combination of clinical features and detection of the c.1824C>T (p.Gly608Gly) heterozygous *LMNA* pathogenic variant, atypical HGPS is diagnosed in individuals who have similar clinical features similar and a progerin-producing pathogenic variant in intron 11 of the *LMNA* gene.

Reference(s): Gordon et al. [100]; Merideth et al. [101].

4.45. Peroxisomal

Testing plasma levels of very long-chain fatty acids (VLCFA) is a common way to screen for certain peroxisomal disorders, though not all patients with peroxisomal disorders have elevated VLCFA. Peroxisomal conditions include, according to one classification scheme, peroxisome biogenesis disorders (Zellweger syndrome, Neonatal adrenoleukodystrophy, Infantile Refsum disease, and Rhizomelic chondrodysplasia punctata), single peroxisomal enzyme deficiencies (such as D-bifunctional protein deficiency), and X-linked adrenoleukodystrophy, which is a peroxisomal substrate transport deficiency. Peroxisomal conditions can affect multiple organ systems and can have a wide spectrum of severity and range of effects. The specific type of peroxisomal disorder may be identified by further biochemical and/or molecular testing beyond VLCFA. There are over a dozen known genes associated with these conditions. Most are inherited in an autosomal recessive manner; X-linked adrenoleukodystrophy is an exception and is also the most common peroxisomal disorder.

Reference(s): Aubourg and Wanders [102]; Steinberg et al. [103].

4.46. *NBN*

Biallelic variants in *NBN* cause Nijmegen breakage syndrome, a condition that can involve intrauterine growth restriction, short stature, progressive microcephaly and intellectual disability, frequent infections, cancer susceptibility, and primary ovarian insufficiency. Heterozygous pathogenic variants have been implicated as causing an increased risk of breast cancer in women and prostate cancer in men, as well as melanoma, and non-Hodgkin lymphoma.

Reference(s): Seemanová et al. [104]; Varon et al. [105].

4.47. C4

Some fatty acid oxidation disorders can be detected by biochemical assays such as on newborn screening or through plasma acylcarnitines due to elevated C4 acylcarnitine. These include Ethylmalonic encephalopathy, Multiple acyl CoA dehydrogenase deficiency, Glutaric acidemia types IIA, IIB, and IIC, Isobutyryl CoA dehydrogenase deficiency, and Short-chain Acyl CoA dehydrogenase deficiency. Other fatty acid oxidation disorders may be detected by different signatures detected through this type of testing.

Reference(s): Rinaldo et al. [106]; American College of Medical Genetics and Genomics ACT Sheets and Confirmatory Algorithms [27].

4.48. *GNAS*

McCune-Albright syndrome is caused by somatic pathogenic variants in the *GNAS* gene. These activating variants occur postzygotically early in embryogenesis. The condition affects multiple organ systems, including the endocrine system, skin, and skeleton. Endocrine manifestations can include acromegaly, growth-hormone secreting pituitary adenomas, hyperparathyroidism, hyperprolactinemia, hyperthyroidism, and precocious puberty. Skin findings include cafeau-lait macules with jagged borders that follow the lines of Blaschko. Skeletal findings primarily involve fibrous dysplasia and can affect multiple bones.

Reference(s): Boyce and Collins [107]; Jones et al. [40].

4.49. Isotretinoin

Isoretinoin/retinoic acid is a medication used to treat acne. Fetal exposure can cause a condition termed retinoic acid embryopathy or fetal retinoid syndrome. This can affect several organ systems, including the craniofacial, cardiovascular, central nervous systems, and can cause other anomalies, such as abnormal thymic development.

Reference(s): Lammer et al. [108]; Jones et al. [40].

4.50. Mitochondria

All of the listed conditions (Alpers-Huttenlocher syndrome, Kearns-Sayre syndrome, Leigh syndrome, Mitochondrial encephalomyopathy, lactic acidosis, and stroke-like episodes (MELAS), and Myoclonic epilepsy with ragged-red fibers (MERFF)) are examples of mitochondrial disorders. Mitochondrial disorders can result from genetic changes affecting the nuclear or mitochondrial DNA. The conditions can involve diverse end-organ effects, and may, depending on the condition, clinically affect one or multiple organ systems.

Reference(s): Gorman et al. [109]; Chinnery [110].

4.51. *SCN5A*

Multiple genes have been implicated in Brugada syndrome, a cardiac arrhythmia syndrome that involves risk of sudden death. Re-evaluation of variants has called certain genes and variants into question in terms of causation, but the *SCN5A* gene is the most frequently involved gene in individuals with Brugada syndrome.

Reference(s): Brugada et al. [111]; Hosseini et al. [112]; Walsh et al. [113].

Chapter 4

4.52. 47,XXY

Klinefelter syndrome most commonly results from the presence of at least one extra X chromosome in addition to the typical 46,XY karyotype. The most common karyotype result in a person considered to have Klinefelter syndrome is 47,XXY. Other karyotypes, such as 48,XXXY, may be observed less commonly in individuals who have more pronounced clinical manifestations of Klinefelter syndrome. Additionally, mosaicism may be observed in some patients. Clinical features of Klinefelter syndrome can be highly variable, and can include increased height, learning and behavioral effects, genitourinary differences (typically mild), and delayed puberty.

Reference(s): Visootsak and Graham [114]; Jones et al. [40].

4.53. 21-hydroxylase

Congenital adrenal hyperplasia (CAH) is a group of conditions that affect the development and function of the adrenal glands. CAH causes impaired steroidogenesis, resulting in the deficient cortisol production that causes clinical manifestations. The most common cause of CAH is 21-hydroxylase deficiency (21-OHD), an autosomal recessive disorder due to biallelic pathogenic variants in *CYP21A2*. Pathogenic variants in other genes can also cause CAH. There are multiple clinical types of 21-OHD, ranging from life-threatening neonatal forms to conditions that are typically not identified until adulthood. Management depends on the type of condition, but early diagnosis is especially critical for some forms.

Reference(s): Nimkarn et al. [115]; El-Maouche et al. [116].

4.54. *SMARCA4, SMARCB1*

Atypical teratoid/rhabdoid tumor (ATRT) is a type of neoplasm of the brain and spinal cord. ATRT most commonly occur in children younger than 3 years of age, but can affect older individuals as well. Pathogenic variants in the tumor suppressor genes *SMARCA4* or *SMARCB1* can result in ATRT as well as predisposition to other rhabdoid tumors.

Reference(s): Frühwald et al. [117]; Nemes et al. [118].

4.55. *GLI3*

Heterozygous pathogenic variants in *GLI3* can cause Grieg cephalopolysyndactyly syndrome (GCPS) or Pallister-Hall syndrome (PHS). "Typical" GCPS can include macrocephaly, hypertelorism, and preaxial polydactyly or mixed pre/postaxial polydactyly; patients may also present with milder or more severe findings. PHS can involve polydactyly, bifid epiglottis, and hypothalamic hamartoma, but can manifest in a much more severe form with laryngotracheal cleft and neonatal lethality.

Reference(s): Johnston et al. [119]; Biesecker [120]; Biesecker and Johnston [121].

4.56. 50%

Fetal cystic hygromas result from abnormal lymphatic development. These can occur anywhere in the body but most commonly affect the head and neck. About 50% of first trimester-affected fetuses will have chromosomal anomalies that are identifiable by karyotype, including aneuploidies affecting chromosomes 13, 18, 21, and the X chromosome, as well as others. In addition to cystic hygroma, other major anomalies are observed in about 30% of fetuses with normal karyotypes.

Reference(s): Malone et al. [122]; Scholl et al. [123]; Stevenson et al. [124].

4.57. *ZEB2*

Mowat-Wilson syndrome is an autosomal dominant disorder caused by heterozygous pathogenic variants in the gene *ZEB2*. The condition can have a wide range of effects, including relating to the severity of disease. Features may include developmental delay/intellectual disability, seizures, microcephaly and distinctive facial features, Hirschsprung disease, and a variety of congenital anomalies that can affect the brain, cardiac, genitourinary, ophthalmologic, and other organ systems.

Reference(s): Garavelli and Mainardi [125]; Ivanovski et al. [126]; Jones et al. [40].

4.58. Diabetes insipidus

Nephrogenic diabetes insipidus may be caused by pathogenic variants in *AVPR2* (X-linked inheritance) or *AQP2* (autosomal dominant or autosomal recessive inheritance). The condition results in inability to concentrate the urine and may manifest with polyuria and polydipsia. In infants, the condition may present with difficulty feeding and voiding, and with failure to thrive and poor activity. The condition can be life-threatening if not diagnosed and treated appropriately related to fluid and electrolyte management.

Reference(s): Bockenhauer and Bichet [127].

4.59. Lesch-Nyhan syndrome

Lesch-Nyhan syndrome is the term given for severe deficiency of the hypoxanthine-guanine phosophoribosyltransferase enzyme, which is caused by pathogenic variants in the gene *HPRT1*. The condition, which is X-linked, typically includes neurologic dysfunction described as resembling cerebral palsy, often with self-injurious behavior, and uric acid overproduction. Neurological findings are usually observed by 3–6 months of age. Less severe forms of disease caused by milder variants in the *HPRT1* gene have also been described.

Reference(s): Torres and Puig [128]; Jinnah [129].

4.60. *PHOX2B*

Congenital central hypoventilation syndrome (CCHS) manifests with autonomic nervous system dysfunction and hypoventilation. There are different forms of the CCHS, including a classic form that presents in infancy, and later-onset forms. The most frequently identified pathogenic variants involve the *PHOX2B* gene. Accurate diagnosis is critical for appropriate management.

Reference(s): Weese-Mayer et al. [130]; Weese-Mayer et al. [131].

4.61. Warfarin

Fetal warfarin syndrome, or Warfarin embryopathy, results from in utero exposure to warfarin. The condition can affect multiple organ systems, but the most frequent findings include nasal hypoplasia and stippling of vertebrae or bony epiphyses.

Reference(s): Basu et al. [132]; Ferreira et al. [133]; Sousa et al. [134].

4.62. *APOE*

Early-onset familial Alzheimer disease (AD) refers to AD that occurs with a mean onset before 65 years of age in multiple members of a family. The clinical condition is otherwise similar to late-onset AD, though can have a long prodromal phase. Pathogenic variants in the genes *APP*, *PSEN1*, and PSEN2 can result in autosomal dominant early-onset familial AD. Variants in the *APOE* gene and in many other genes (as well as nongenetic factors) may also contribute to a person's susceptibility to AD.

Reference(s): Schellenberg and Montine [135]; Cacace et al. [136]; Bird [137].

4.63. All of the above

People of Ashkenazi Jewish ancestry are more likely to carry pathogenic variants related to a number of conditions. Examples of these conditions include Bloom syndrome, Canavan disease, Cystic fibrosis, Familial dysautonomia, Fanconi anemia group C, GD, Mucolipidosis IV, Niemann-Pick disease, type A, and Tay-Sachs disease. There are also other conditions that are more common in people of this ancestry. People of other ancestries may also be more likely to carry pathogenic variants related to other (or the same) genetic conditions.

Reference(s): Zhang et al. [138]; Rose and Wick [139]; King and Klugman [140].

4.64. *APOL1*

Many genetic and nongenetic factors may contribute to kidney disease. Specific variants in the gene *APOL1* are associated with risk of a type of chronic kidney disease known as Focal segmental glomerulosclerosis (FSGS). *APOL1* can relate to other clinical situations as well – for example, there appear to be effects on the efficacy of renal transplant based on donor *APOL1* status. Variants in *APOL1* also seem to explain at least part of why people from certain ancestries may be more prone to kidney disease.

Reference(s): Rosenberg and Kopp [141]; Freedman et al. [142]; Kopp and Winkler [143].

4.65. *KMT2D* and *KDM6A*

Kabuki syndrome is a genetic disorder that involves distinctive facial features, skeletal anomalies, persistent fetal fingertip pads, intellectual disability, and growth deficiency, as well as other features, including congenital malformations affecting the heart and gastrointestinal system. Kabuki syndrome can be caused by pathogenic variants in the *KMT2D* or *KDM6A* genes.

Reference(s): Adam et al. [144]; Adam et al. [145]; Jones et al. [40].

4.66. Can screen for aneuploidies and other conditions

Noninvasive prenatal screening (NIPS), sometimes called noninvasive prenatal testing (NIPT), screens for certain fetal genetic disorders that can be assessed through a peripheral blood sample taken from the pregnant mother. Depending on the specific testing approach, aneuploidies affecting chromosomes 13, 18, 21, X, and Y are examined; other aneuploidies and other conditions, such as those due to specific missing or extra portions of DNA may also be examined.

Reference(s): Bianchi and Wilkins-Haug [146]; Committee on Practice Bulletins [147]; Taylor-Phillips et al. [148].

4.67. 50–100

In 2013, the American College of Medical Genetics and Genomics (ACMG) published a minimum list of 56 genes to be reported as incidental or secondary findings in the context of clinical genomic (exome or genome) sequencing. The goal was to encourage standardized reporting of actionable information for certain conditions in order to allow interventions that would prevent or reduce morbidity and mortality. Through ongoing efforts, a revised policy statement in 2017 removed one of these genes and added four more, such that 59 such genes were listed. The 2021 revision included 73 genes. Other entities, such as European societies, have different interpretations and lists.

Reference(s): Green et al. [149]; Kalia et al. [150]; Miller et al. [151].

4.68. Tyrosinemia type I

Tyrosinemia type I is an autosomal recessive biochemical disorder caused by deficiency of the enzyme fumarylacetoacetase (FAH). The condition results from biallelic pathogenic variants in *FAH*. If not identified via newborn screening (due to detection of succinylacetone) and treated, the condition may present with severe hepatic dysfunction, renal tubular dysfunction with growth failure and rickets, and with episodic neurologic crises.

Reference(s): Chinsky et al. [152].

4.69. Keratin

There are over 50 known functional keratin genes in humans, which are divided into two main groups. These genes encode keratin proteins, which serve multiple cellular mechanisms in epithelial cells. Pathogenic variants in the keratin genes can lead to multiple conditions in humans, including Epidermolysis bullosa, Pachyonychia congenita, and forms of ichthyosis, as well as other disorders.

Reference(s): Lane and McLean [153]; Irvine [154]; Jacob et al. [155].

4.70. *TP63*

Pathogenic variants in the *TP63* gene can result in a number of phenotypes, including Acro-dermo-ungual-lacrimal-tooth (ADULT) syndrome; Ankyloblepharon-ectodermal defects-cleft lip/palate (AEC) syndrome/Rapp-Hodgkin syndrome; Ectrodactyly, ectodermal dysplasia, cleft lip/palate syndrome; Isolated cleft lip/cleft palate; Limb-mammary syndrome; Split-hand/foot malformation. Individual syndromes have specific findings, but common manifestations may include cleft lip/palate, ectodermal dysplasia (dental and nail anomalies, sparse hair, and hypohidrosis), hypopigmentation, hypoplastic breasts and/or nipples, lacrimal duct obstruction, and split-hand/foot malformations/syndactyly. Features may differ significantly between patients, including within individual families.

Reference(s): Eisenkraft et al. [156]; Wenger et al. [157]; Sutton and van Bokhoven [158].

4.71. Karyotype

There are a number of well-characterized microdeletion syndromes, which by definition involve submicroscopic chromosomal deletions. Deletions at least 5 Mb in size are usually visible by karyotype, such that a routine karyotype would not be expected to reliably detect the genetic change described in this case. Other methods, such as targeted fluorescence in situ hybridization (FISH) testing, microarray, or exome sequencing with reliable copy number variant (CNV) calling, should all be able to confirm the genetic diagnosis.

Reference(s): Jones et al. [40].

4.72. *CDC73*

Heterozygous pathogenic variants in *CDC73* can cause conditions such as Hyperparathyrodism-jaw tumor (HPT-JT) syndrome, CDC73-related parathyroid carcinoma, and Familial isolated hyperparathyroidism. HPT-JT involves hyperparathyrodism, which is usually due to a parathyroid adenoma, as well as jaw fibromas; the condition can also include other types of neoplasms as well as manifestations like kidney cysts.

Reference(s): Cardoso et al. [159]; van der Tuin et al. [160]; Hyde et al. [161].

4.73. Somatic

One type of tumor-based genetic testing, sometimes called somatic cancer testing, can be used to evaluate a neoplasm for genetic changes that may help better understand factors such as the specific tumor subtype, prognosis, and therapeutic options. Genetic variants identified in the tumor sample may have arisen in the tumor itself – this is a type of somatic variant. However, somatic variants can occur outside the context of cancer. In the example in the question, testing has shown that the somatic variant does not appear to be present in the rest of the person's DNA. On the other hand, it is possible that a genetic change observed in a tumor could represent a germline or constitutional change, where the genetic change is present in the person's other, non-tumor cells.

Reference(s): Raymond et al. [162]; Uzilov et al. [163]; Li et al. [164].

4.74. Becker muscular dystrophy and Duchenne muscular dystrophy

Becker muscular dystrophy (BMD) and Duchenne muscular dystrophy (DMD) are X-linked genetic conditions caused by pathogenic variants in the *DMD* gene. Changes in this gene can also cause DMD-associated cardiomyopathy. Conditions related to this gene, which are sometimes called Dystrophinopathies, are considered a spectrum of disease. DMD often manifests in early childhood with calf hypertrophy, motor developmental delay, proximal weakness, waddling gait, and a very high level of serum creatine phosphokinase (CK); later, respiratory and cardiac complications may occur. BMD often presents with later and milder findings.

Reference(s): Flanigan [165]; Aartsma-Rus et al. [166]; Darras et al. [167].

4.75. Prostate cancer

Most cases of prostate cancer appear to develop sporadically, but approximately 10% or more cases of prostate cancer have been reported to be due to identifiable, hereditary predisposition. Variants in multiple genes may result in hereditary predisposition to prostate cancer. Among these, specific pathogenic variants in the gene *HOXB13* have been shown to result in an increased risk of prostate cancer.

Reference(s): Ewing et al. [168]; Dias et al. [169]; Giri et al. [170]; Zhen et al. [171].

4.76. *HMBS*

Acute intermittent porphyria (AIP) is an autosomal dominant condition caused by pathogenic variants in *HMBS*, which encodes the enzyme hydroxymethylbilane synthase. The condition involves attacks of acute abdominal pain, which may be accompanied by other signs and symptoms, including neurologic findings. There are also other genetic forms of porphyria. Accurate and timely diagnosis can be important for optimal care.

Reference(s): Wang et al. [172]; Bonkovsky et al. [173]; Whatley and Badminton [174].

4.77. Amino acidemia

There are many types of inborn errors of metabolism (IEM). These are often grouped according to the underlying biochemical/biologic features related to the diseases. Amino acidemias, or amino acid metabolism disorders, involve abnormalities in the metabolism of amino acids. Buildup of specific amino acids caused by these IEM can result in adverse health effects. Examples of amino acidemias include Arginenemia, Maple syrup urine disease, Phenylketonuria, and Tyrosinemia, as well as other conditions such as Arginosuccinic aciduria, Citrullinemia, and Homocystinuria.

Reference(s): Burton [175]; Levy [176].

4.78. *BMPR1A*

In 2013, the American College of Medical Genetics and Genomics (ACMG) published a list of genes in which relevant results are recommended to be reported as incidental or secondary findings when identified through clinical genomic (exome or genome) sequencing. More recent policy statements continue to revise these lists. These genes are associated with different conditions affecting various organ systems, including genes involved in biochemical, cardiovascular, oncologic, and other disorders. Among the genes included, pathogenic variants in *BMPR1A* cause Juvenile polypsosis syndrome, which involves a predisposition to GI polyps, in which malignant transformation can occur. Diagnosis is important for optimal clinical management.

Reference(s): Green et al. [149]; Haidle and Howe [177]; Kalia et al. [150].

4.79. Exons

There are thousands of genetic conditions for which causes have been identified. The application of technologies such as exome and genome sequencing has greatly accelerated the ability to provide molecular diagnoses for affected patients (and to find new, molecular explanations for many disorders of previously unknown etiology). To date, the majority of pathogenic variants that cause these conditions have been identified as being located in the exons. This may reflect the importance of the exons related to human disease, as well as the fact that the exons have been investigated more extensively than other regions of the genome.

References: Boycott et al. [178]; Clark et al. [179]; Short et al. [180]; Bamshad et al. [181]; Wells et al. [182].

4.80. *HTRA1*

Variants in multiple genes have been reported as associated with monogenic forms of Parkinson disease (PD). Implicated genes include *GBA*, *LRRK2*, and *PRKN*, which are associated with adult-onset forms. Other genes have also been implicated in PD, including adult and pediatric-onset forms. In addition to these monogenic conditions, other genes and loci have been identified through genome-wide association studies. However, the cause(s) of PD remain unknown in most patients.

Reference(s): Lunati et al. [183].

4.81. Human leukocyte antigen

The major histocompatibility complex (MHC) is a group of genes found in many different species. The human histocompatibility complex (the human version of the MHC complex) is called the human leukocyte antigen (HLA) complex. This includes over 200 genes, which are found on chromosome 6. There are different groups, or classes, of HLA genes; the nomenclature used to describe these genes and their variants is different from that of other genes and variants. The HLA complex helps the immune system distinguish the body's own proteins from foreign proteins.

Reference(s): Marsh et al. [184]; Dendrou et al. [185].

4.82. *ANK1*

Hereditary spherocytosis can manifest with anemia, jaundice, and splenomegaly. Pathogenic variants in *ANK1*, as well as several other genes, can cause hereditary spherocytosis. Diagnosis is important to manage sequelae of the disease, such as through blood transfusions, which may be required (among other interventions).

Reference(s): Eber et al. [186]; Tole et al. [187].

4.83. Complete

Molar pregnancies involve aberrant growth of trophoblast cells, which normally develop into the placenta. In a complete molar pregnancy, all the genetic material is from the father because an "empty" egg is fertilized by one or two sperm. In a partial molar pregnancy, an egg containing the mother's genetic material is fertilized (most often) by two sperm. Molar pregnancy can involve risk of progression to a type of cancer called choriocarcinoma; this is more common in complete molar pregnancies.

Reference(s): Eagles et al. [188]; Hui et al. [189]; Nguyen et al. [190].

4.84. *PTEN*

Some "inherited cancer syndromes" include features that may help suggest a specific inherited/germline cause. "PTEN hamartoma tumor syndrome" (PHTS) refers to a group of conditions that include entities known as Cowden syndrome (CS), and Bannayan-Riley-Ruvalcaba syndrome (BRRS), as well as other conditions with overlapping features. CS (as more classically defined) includes macrocephaly, skin findings such as trichilemmomas and papillomatous papules, and increased risk for breast, endometrial, and thyroid tumors.

Reference(s): Nagy et al. [191]; Yehia and Eng [192].

4.85. Krabbe disease

Krabbe disease results from deficiency of the enzyme galactocerebrosidase. The condition can manifest in infancy or later in life (earlier-onset forms appear more common). In infancy, signs of Krabbe disease can include irritability, spasticity, and other signs of neurocognitive sequelae such as developmental delay. Krabbe disease results from biallelic pathogenic variants in *GALC*.

Reference(s): Kwon et al. [193]; Orsini et al. [194]; Komatsuzaki et al. [195].

4.86. Collagen

Pathogenic variants in the collagen genes can result in a number of different conditions. An important group of conditions that can be caused by pathogenic variants in these genes are certain skeletal dysplasias (skeletal dysplasias can also be caused by changes in other genes). Examples of skeletal conditions that involve collagen genes include some types of Osteogenesis imperfecta.

Reference(s): Lachman et al. [196]; Besio et al. [197]; Marini and Do [198].

4.87. Duarte

In Duarte variant galactosemia, the activity of the enzyme erythrocyte galactose-1-phosphate uridylyltransferase (GALT) is about 25% of normal. In individuals with this finding from biochemically based laboratory testing, molecular testing of the *GALT* gene usually shows one pathogenic GALT variant and heterozygosity or homozygosity for the genetic variant resulting in the Duarte biochemical finding. Current evidence indicates that infants with Duarte variant galactosemia who are fed with breast milk or dairy milk-based formula are usually asymptomatic, with the same prevalence of acute medical issues as the general infant population.

Reference(s): Feuchtbaum et al. [199]; Fridovich-Keil et al. [200].

4.88. Achondroplasia

In general, certain genetic conditions can be due to inherited or de novo pathogenic. According to the literature, about 80% of individuals with Achondroplasia, 25% of individuals with Marfan syndrome, 50% of individuals with Neurofibromatosis type 1, and 67% of individuals with Tuberous sclerosis complex (TSC) have the condition due to de novo pathogenic variants (versus variants inherited from a parent), respectively.

Reference(s): Wilkin et al. [201]; Acuna-Hidalgo et al. [202]; Dietz [203]; Friedman [204]; Legare [205]; Northrup et al. [206].

4.89. RASopathy

The term "RASopathy" refers to a group of genetic conditions that can be caused by pathogenic variants in genes involved in the RAS-mitogen activated protein kinase (MAPK) pathway. Pathogenic variants in multiple known genes can cause RASopathies, with more such genes continuing to be identified. RASopathies include Cardio-Facio-Cutaneous syndrome; Costello syndrome; Legius syndrome; Neurofibromatosis type 1; Noonan syndrome. The conditions affect multiple organ systems, and the various conditions can involve overlapping features.

Reference(s): Allanson and Roberts [20]; Gripp et al. [207]; Gross et al. [208].

4.90. *TBX1*

TBX1, a member of a conserved gene family that shares a common DNA-binding domain (the T-box), is located on chromosome 22q11.2. Pathogenic variants in this gene can result in at least some of the manifestations of 22q11.2 deletion syndrome.

Reference(s): Jerome and Papaioannou [209]; Yagi et al. [210]; Paylor et al. [211]; Zweier et al. [212].

4.91. Proteus syndrome

Genetic conditions can be caused by pathogenic variants that are inherited, or which arise at various stages of development and life. The affected gene, the timing of the variant (when during development or life the variant occurs), and the tissue(s) affected influence the disease type and course. Proteus syndrome is an overgrowth disorder caused by somatic activating variants in *AKT1*.

Reference(s): Lindhurst et al. [213]; Levy-Lahad and King [214].

4.92. Urine glycosaminoglycans

"Coarse" facial features is a historical term used to describe thickened skin (with or without thickening of the underlying tissues) or more rounded facial

Chapter 4

features, and generally refers to a less sharp appearance of the facial structures. This finding can occur in a number of different genetic conditions, including mucopolysaccharidoses, of which there are multiple different types. In a patient with a suspected mucopolysaccharidosis, the diagnostic process can include testing of urinary glycosaminoglycans (GAGs) as an initial part of the overall workup. Accurate diagnosis (including via more specific testing modalities than urinary GAGs) can be important to ensure precise diagnosis and medical management.

Reference(s): Lawrence et al. [215]; Kubaski et al. [216]; National Human Genome Research Institute, [217].

4.93. 45,X

Turner syndrome occurs due to the absence of all or part of one copy of the X chromosome. About half of people with Turner syndrome have monosomy X (which is written as 45,X, not 45,XO). Approximately 10% of individuals with Turner syndrome have a duplication (isochromosome) of the long arm of one of the X chromosomes. Most of the rest of people with Turner syndrome will have mosaicism for 45,X along with the presence of additional cell lineages, such as 46,XX.

Reference(s): Ranke and Saenger [218]; Kruszka and Silberbach [219]; San Roman and Page [220].

4.94. *MET*

MET is a protooncogene; heterozygous pathogenic variants in this gene have been described in Hereditary papillary renal cell carcinoma, a type of hereditary renal cancer. Hereditary renal cancer may also occur related to variants in other genes, such as *FH*, *FLCN*, *VHL*, and others; cytogenomic abnormalities may also contribute to oncogenesis. In addition to Hereditary papillary renal cell carcinoma, variants in the *MET* gene may also result in other genetic conditions.

Reference(s): Zhuang et al. [221]; Yang et al. [222]; Dizman et al. [223].

4.95. Steroid sulfatase

Steroid sulfatase deficiency, which results from pathogenic variants affecting *STS*, is an X-linked condition sometimes referred to as X-linked ichthyosis. The condition can also include corneal opacities, cryptorchidism, and neurological manifestations. There are many other genetic conditions that also cause ichthyosis.

Reference(s): Hernández-Martín et al. [224]; Fischer and Bourrat [225].

References

1. Kaurah, P. and Huntsman, D.G. (1993). Hereditary diffuse gastric cancer. In: *GeneReviews®* (ed. M.P. Adam, H.H. Ardinger, R.A. Pagon, et al.). Seattle, WA: University of Washington.
2. van der Post, R.S., Vogelaar, I.P., Carneiro, F. et al. (2015). Hereditary diffuse gastric cancer: updated clinical guidelines with an emphasis on germline CDH1 mutation carriers. *J. Med. Genet.* 52: 361–374.
3. Petrovchich, I. and Ford, J.M. (2016). Genetic predisposition to gastric cancer. *Semin. Oncol.* 43: 554–559.

4. Bagni, C., Tassone, F., Neri, G., and Hagerman, R. (2012). Fragile X syndrome: causes, diagnosis, mechanisms, and therapeutics. *J. Clin. Invest.* 122: 4314–4322.

5. Hunter, J.E., Berry-Kravis, E., Hipp, H., and Todd, P.K. (1993). FMR1 disorders. In: *GeneReviews*® (ed. M.P. Adam, H.H. Ardinger, R.A. Pagon, et al.). Seattle, WA: University of Washington.

6. Leiding, J.W. and Holland, S.M. (1993). Chronic granulomatous disease. In: *GeneReviews*® (ed. M.P. Adam, H.H. Ardinger, R.A. Pagon, et al.). Seattle, WA: University of Washington.

7. Arnold, D.E. and Heimall, J.R. (2017). A review of chronic granulomatous disease. *Adv. Ther.* 34: 2543–2557.

8. Manasse, B.F., Lekgate, N., Pfaffenzeller, W.M., and de Ravel, T.J. (2000). The Pallister-Killian syndrome is reliably diagnosed by FISH on buccal mucosa. *Clin. Dysmorphol.* 9: 163–165.

9. Karaman, B., Kayserili, H., Ghanbari, A. et al. (2018). Pallister-Killian syndrome: clinical, cytogenetic and molecular findings in 15 cases. *Mol. Cytogenet.* 11: 45.

10. Bertini, V., Gana, S., Orsini, A. et al. (2019). Advantages of array comparative genomic hybridization using buccal swab DNA for detecting Pallister-Killian syndrome. *Ann. Lab. Med.* 39: 232–234.

11. Leongamornlert, D., Saunders, E., Dadaev, T. et al. (2014). Frequent germline deleterious mutations in DNA repair genes in familial prostate cancer cases are associated with advanced disease. *Br. J. Cancer* 110: 1663–1672.

12. Mateo, J., Carreira, S., Sandhu, S. et al. (2015). DNA-repair defects and olaparib in metastatic prostate cancer. *N. Engl. J. Med.* 373: 1697–1708.

13. Pritchard, C.C., Mateo, J., Walsh, M.F. et al. (2016). Inherited DNA-repair gene mutations in men with metastatic prostate cancer. *N. Engl. J. Med.* 375: 443–453.

14. Giri, V.N., Hegarty, S.E., Hyatt, C. et al. (2019). Germline genetic testing for inherited prostate cancer in practice: Implications for genetic testing, precision therapy, and cascade testing. *Prostate* 79: 333–339.

15. Wilch, E.S. and Morton, C.C. (2018). Historical and clinical perspectives on chromosomal translocations. *Adv. Exp. Med. Biol.* 1044: 1–14.

16. Nussbaum, R.L., McInnes, R.R., and Willard, H.F. (2016). *Thompson & Thompson Genetics in Medicine*. Philadelphia, PA: Elsevier.

17. Stoller, J.K. and Aboussouan, L.S. (2005). Alpha1-antitrypsin deficiency. *Lancet* 365: 2225–2236.

18. Greene, C.M., Marciniak, S.J., Teckman, J. et al. (2016). Alpha1-antitrypsin deficiency. *Nat. Rev. Dis. Primers.* 2: 16051.

19. Stoller, J.K., Hupertz, V., and Aboussouan, L.S. (1993). Alpha-1 antitrypsin deficiency. In: *GeneReviews*® (ed. M.P. Adam, H.H. Ardinger, R.A. Pagon, et al.). Seattle, WA: University of Washington.

20. Allanson, J.E. and Roberts, A.E. (1993). Noonan syndrome. In: *GeneReviews*® (ed. M.P. Adam, H.H. Ardinger, R.A. Pagon, et al.). Seattle, WA: University of Washington.

21. Liao, J. and Mehta, L. (2019). Molecular genetics of Noonan syndrome and RASopathies. *Pediatr. Endocrinol. Rev.* 16: 435–446.

22. Biesecker, L.G. and Green, R.C. (2014). Diagnostic clinical genome and exome sequencing. *N. Engl. J. Med.* 370: 2418–2425.

Chapter 4

23. Driscoll, D.J., Miller, J.L., Schwartz, S., and Cassidy, S.B. (1993). Prader-Willi syndrome. In: *GeneReviews*® (ed. M.P. Adam, H.H. Ardinger, R.A. Pagon, et al.). Seattle, WA: University of Washington.

24. Helbig, I. and Tayoun, A.A. (2016). Understanding genotypes and phenotypes in epileptic encephalopathies. *Mol. Syndromol.* 7 (4): 172–181. https://doi.org/10.1159/000448530. Epub 2016 Aug 20. PMID: 27781027; PMCID: PMC5073622.

25. Miller, I.O. and Sotero de Menezes, M.A. (2007 Nov 29 [updated 2022 Feb 17]). SCN1A seizure disorders. In: *GeneReviews*® *[Internet]* (ed. M.P. Adam, H.H. Ardinger, R.A. Pagon, et al.). Seattle, WA: University of Washington, Seattle; 1993–2022. PMID: 20301494.

26. Wheless, J.W., Fulton, S.P., and Mudigoudar, B.D. (2020). Dravet syndrome: a review of current management. *Pediatr. Neurol.* 107: 28–40.

27. Newborn screening ACT sheets and algorithms. https://www.ncbi.nlm.nih.gov/books/NBK55827/ (accessed 26 July 21.).

28. HRSA recommended uniform screening panel. https://www.hrsa.gov/advisorycommittees/mchbadvisory/heritabledisorders/recommendedpanel/ (accessed 26 July 21).

29. McBride, K.A., Ballinger, M.L., Killick, E. et al. (2014). Li-Fraumeni syndrome: cancer risk assessment and clinical management. *Nat. Rev. Clin. Oncol.* 11: 260–271.

30. Schneider, K., Zelley, K., Nichols, K.E., and Garber, J. (1993). Li-Fraumeni syndrome. In: *GeneReviews*® (ed. M.P. Adam, H.H. Ardinger, R.A. Pagon, et al.). Seattle, WA: University of Washington.

31. Ironside, J.W., Ritchie, D.L., and Head, M.W. (2017). Prion diseases. *Handb. Clin. Neurol.* 145: 393–403.

32. Tee, B.L., Longoria Ibarrola, E.M., and Geschwind, M.D. (2018). Prion diseases. *Neurol. Clin.* 36: 865–897.

33. Zerr, I. and Schmitz, M. (1993). Genetic prion disease. In: *GeneReviews*® (ed. M.P. Adam, H.H. Ardinger, R.A. Pagon, et al.). Seattle, WA: University of Washington.

34. Hall, B.D., Cadle, R.G., Morrill-Cornelius, S.M., and Bay, C.A. (2007). Phakomatosis pigmentovascularis: implications for severity with special reference to Mongolian spots associated with Sturge-Weber and Klippel-Trenaunay syndromes. *Am. J. Med. Genet. A* 143A: 3047–3053.

35. Ch'ng, S. and Tan, S.T. (2008). Facial port-wine stains – clinical stratification and risks of neuro-ocular involvement. *J. Plast. Reconstr. Aesthet. Surg.* 61: 889–893.

36. Piram, M., Lorette, G., Sirinelli, D. et al. (2012). Sturge-Weber syndrome in patients with facial port-wine stain. *Pediatr. Dermatol.* 29: 32–37.

37. Shirley, M.D., Tang, H., Gallione, C.J. et al. (2013). Sturge-Weber syndrome and port-wine stains caused by somatic mutation in GNAQ. *N. Engl. J. Med.* 368: 1971–1979.

38. Foster, A., Zachariou, A., Loveday, C. et al. (2019). The phenotype of Sotos syndrome in adulthood: a review of 44 individuals. *Am. J. Med. Genet. C Semin. Med. Genet.* 181: 502–508.

39. Tatton-Brown, K., Cole, T.R.P., and Rahman, N. (1993). Sotos syndrome. In: *GeneReviews*® (ed. M.P. Adam, H.H. Ardinger, R.A. Pagon, et al.). Seattle, WA: University of Washington.

40. Jones, K., Jones, M., and del Campo, M. (2021). *Smith's Recognizable Patterns of Human Malformation*. Philadelphia, PA: Elsevier, Inc.

41. Haeusler, A.R., Donnelly, C.J., and Rothstein, J.D. (2016). The expanding biology of the C9orf72 nucleotide repeat expansion in neurodegenerative disease. *Nat. Rev. Neurosci.* 17: 383–395.

42. Gijselinck, I., Cruts, M., and Van Broeckhoven, C. (2018). The Genetics of C9orf72 Expansions. *Cold Spring Harb. Perspect. Med.* 8.

43. Pai, S.Y., Logan, B.R., Griffith, L.M. et al. (2014). Transplantation outcomes for severe combined immunodeficiency, 2000–2009. *N. Engl. J. Med.* 371: 434–446.

44. Kwan, A. and Puck, J.M. (2015). History and current status of newborn screening for severe combined immunodeficiency. *Semin. Perinatol.* 39: 194–205.

45. Sampson, J.R., Dolwani, S., Jones, S. et al. (2003). Autosomal recessive colorectal adenomatous polyposis due to inherited mutations of MYH. *Lancet* 362: 39–41.

46. Wimmer, K. and Kratz, C.P. (2010). Constitutional mismatch repair-deficiency syndrome. *Haematologica* 95: 699–701.

47. Nielsen, M., Infante, E., and Brand, R. (1993). MUTYH polyposis. In: *GeneReviews®* (ed. M.P. Adam, H.H. Ardinger, R.A. Pagon, et al.). Seattle, WA: University of Washington.

48. Piel, F.B., Steinberg, M.H., and Rees, D.C. (2017). Sickle cell disease. *N. Engl. J. Med.* 376: 1561–1573.

49. Bender, M.A. (1993). Sickle cell disease. In: *GeneReviews®* (ed. M.P. Adam, H.H. Ardinger, R.A. Pagon, et al.). Seattle, WA: University of Washington.

50. Slager, R.E., Newton, T.L., Vlangos, C.N. et al. (2003). Mutations in RAI1 associated with Smith-Magenis syndrome. *Nat. Genet.* 33: 466–468.

51. Smith, A.C.M., Boyd, K.E., Brennan, C. et al. (1993). Smith-Magenis syndrome. In: *GeneReviews®* (ed. M.P. Adam, H.H. Ardinger, R.A. Pagon, et al.). Seattle, WA: University of Washington.

52. Neul, J.L., Kaufmann, W.E., Glaze, D.G. et al. (2010). Rett syndrome: revised diagnostic criteria and nomenclature. *Ann. Neurol.* 68: 944–950.

53. Leonard, H., Cobb, S., and Downs, J. (2017). Clinical and biological progress over 50 years in Rett syndrome. *Nat. Rev. Neurol.* 13: 37–51.

54. Kaur, S. and Christodoulou, J. (1993). MECP2 disorders. In: *GeneReviews®* (ed. M.P. Adam, H.H. Ardinger, R.A. Pagon, et al.). Seattle, WA: University of Washington.

55. Ferreira, C.R. and Gahl, W.A. (2017). Disorders of metal metabolism. *Transl. Sci. Rare Dis.* 2: 101–139.

56. Beggs, A.D., Latchford, A.R., Vasen, H.F. et al. (2010). Peutz-Jeghers syndrome: a systematic review and recommendations for management. *Gut* 59: 975–986.

57. McGarrity, T.J., Amos, C.I., and Baker, M.J. (1993). Peutz-Jeghers syndrome. In: *GeneReviews®* (ed. M.P. Adam, H.H. Ardinger, R.A. Pagon, et al.). Seattle, WA: University of Washington.

58. Shapiro, E., Krivit, W., Lockman, L. et al. (2000). Long-term effect of bone-marrow transplantation for childhood-onset cerebral X-linked adrenoleukodystrophy. *Lancet* 356: 713–718.

59. Raymond, G.V., Moser, A.B., and Fatemi, A. (1993). X-linked adrenoleukodystrophy. In: *GeneReviews®* (ed. M.P. Adam, H.H. Ardinger, R.A. Pagon, et al.). Seattle, WA: University of Washington.

60. Tully, H.M. and Dobyns, W.B. (2014). Infantile hydrocephalus: a review of epidemiology, classification and causes. *Eur. J. Med. Genet.* 57: 359–368.

61. Stumpel, C. and Vos, Y.J. (1993). L1 syndrome. In: *GeneReviews®* (ed. M.P. Adam, H.H. Ardinger, R.A. Pagon, et al.). Seattle, WA: University of Washington.

62. Adams, P.C., Reboussin, D.M., Barton, J.C. et al. (2005). Hemochromatosis and iron-overload screening in a racially diverse population. *N. Engl. J. Med.* 352: 1769–1778.

63. Barton, J.C. and Edwards, C.Q. (1993). HFE hemochromatosis. In: *GeneReviews®* (ed. M.P. Adam, H.H. Ardinger, R.A. Pagon, et al.). Seattle, WA: University of Washington.

64. Richards, S., Aziz, N., Bale, S. et al. (2015). Standards and guidelines for the interpretation of sequence variants: a joint consensus recommendation of the American College of Medical Genetics and Genomics and the Association for Molecular Pathology. *Genet. Med.* 17: 405–424.

65. Mersch, J., Brown, N., Pirzadeh-Miller, S. et al. (2018). Prevalence of variant reclassification following hereditary cancer genetic testing. *JAMA* 320: 1266–1274.

66. Deignan, J.L., Chung, W.K., Kearney, H.M. et al. (2019). Points to consider in the reevaluation and reanalysis of genomic test results: a statement of the American College of Medical Genetics and Genomics (ACMG). *Genet. Med.* 21: 1267–1270.

67. Harrison, S.M. and Rehm, H.L. (2019). Is "likely pathogenic" really 90% likely? Reclassification data in ClinVar. *Genome Med.* 11: 72.

68. Schultz, K.A., Yang, J., Doros, L. et al. (2014). DICER1-pleuropulmonary blastoma familial tumor predisposition syndrome: a unique constellation of neoplastic conditions. *Pathol. Case Rev.* 19: 90–100.

69. Schultz, K.A.P., Stewart, D.R., Kamihara, J. et al. (1993). DICER1 tumor predisposition. In: *GeneReviews®* (ed. M.P. Adam, H.H. Ardinger, R.A. Pagon, et al.). Seattle, WA: University of Washington.

70. Mistry, P.K., Lopez, G., Schiffmann, R. et al. (2017). Gaucher disease: progress and ongoing challenges. *Mol. Genet. Metab.* 120: 8–21.

71. Pastores, G.M. and Hughes, D.A. (1993). Gaucher disease. In: *GeneReviews®* (ed. M.P. Adam, H.H. Ardinger, R.A. Pagon, et al.). Seattle, WA: University of Washington.

72. Scheuerle, A.E. and Ursini, M.V. (1993). Incontinentia pigmenti. In: *GeneReviews®* (ed. M.P. Adam, H.H. Ardinger, R.A. Pagon, et al.). Seattle, WA: University of Washington.

73. Rice, G., Patrick, T., Parmar, R. et al. (2007). Clinical and molecular phenotype of Aicardi-Goutieres syndrome. *Am. J. Hum. Genet.* 81: 713–725.

74. Armangue, T., Orsini, J.J., Takanohashi, A. et al. (2017). Neonatal detection of Aicardi Goutieres syndrome by increased C26:0 lysophosphatidylcholine and interferon signature on newborn screening blood spots. *Mol. Genet. Metab.* 122: 134–139.

75. Lee, S., Clinard, K., Young, S.P. et al. (2020). Evaluation of X-linked adrenoleukodystrophy newborn screening in North Carolina. *JAMA Netw. Open* 3: e1920356.

76. Tise, C.G., Morales, J.A., Lee, A.S. et al. (2021). Aicardi-Goutieres syndrome may present with positive newborn screen for X-linked adrenoleukodystrophy. *Am. J. Med. Genet. A* 185: 1848–1853.

77. Hegde, M., Ferber, M., Mao, R. et al. (2014). ACMG technical standards and guidelines for genetic testing for inherited colorectal cancer (Lynch syndrome, familial adenomatous polyposis, and MYH-associated polyposis). *Genet. Med.* 16: 101–116.

78. Idos, G. and Valle, L. (1993). Lynch syndrome. In: *GeneReviews®* (ed. M.P. Adam, H.H. Ardinger, R.A. Pagon, et al.). Seattle, WA: University of Washington.

Chapter 4

79. Ruberg, F.L. and Berk, J.L. (2012). Transthyretin (TTR) cardiac amyloidosis. *Circulation* 126: 1286–1300.

80. Sekijima, Y. (1993). Hereditary transthyretin amyloidosis. In: *GeneReviews*® (ed. M.P. Adam, H.H. Ardinger, R.A. Pagon, et al.). Seattle, WA: University of Washington.

81. Rauen, K.A. (2013). The RASopathies. *Annu. Rev. Genomics Hum. Genet.* 14: 355–369.

82. Legius, E. and Stevenson, D. (1993). Legius syndrome. In: *GeneReviews*® (ed. M.P. Adam, H.H. Ardinger, R.A. Pagon, et al.). Seattle, WA: University of Washington.

83. Flanagan, M. and Cunniff, C.M. (1993). Bloom syndrome. In: *GeneReviews*® (ed. M.P. Adam, H.H. Ardinger, R.A. Pagon, et al.). Seattle, WA: University of Washington.

84. DevCan - probability of developing or dying of cancer. https://surveillance.cancer.gov/devcan/ (accessed 26 July 21).

85. Leachman, S.A., Lucero, O.M., Sampson, J.E. et al. (2017). Identification, genetic testing, and management of hereditary melanoma. *Cancer Metastasis Rev.* 36: 77–90.

86. Vogelstein, B. and Kinzler, K.W. (1999). Digital PCR. *Proc. Natl Acad. Sci. USA* 96: 9236–9241.

87. Lindy, A.S., Stosser, M.B., Butler, E. et al. (2018). Diagnostic outcomes for genetic testing of 70 genes in 8565 patients with epilepsy and neurodevelopmental disorders. *Epilepsia* 59: 1062–1071.

88. Zhou, B., Haney, M.S., Zhu, X. et al. (2018). Detection and quantification of mosaic genomic DNA variation in primary somatic tissues using ddPCR: analysis of mosaic transposable-element insertions, copy-number variants, and single-nucleotide variants. *Methods Mol. Biol.* 1768: 173–190.

89. Beck, D.B., Ferrada, M.A., Sikora, K.A. et al. (2020). Somatic mutations in UBA1 and severe adult-onset autoinflammatory disease. *N. Engl. J. Med.* 383 (27): 2628–2638.

90. Udd, B. and Krahe, R. (2012). The myotonic dystrophies: molecular, clinical, and therapeutic challenges. *Lancet Neurol.* 11: 891–905.

91. Bird, T.D. (1993). Myotonic dystrophy type 1. In: *GeneReviews*® (ed. M.P. Adam, H.H. Ardinger, R.A. Pagon, et al.). Seattle, WA: University of Washington.

92. Ingles, J., Burns, C., Barratt, A., and Semsarian, C. (2015). Application of genetic testing in hypertrophic cardiomyopathy for preclinical disease detection. *Circ. Cardiovasc. Genet.* 8: 852–859.

93. Cirino, A.L. and Ho, C. (1993). Hypertrophic cardiomyopathy overview. In: *GeneReviews*® (ed. M.P. Adam, H.H. Ardinger, R.A. Pagon, et al.). Seattle, WA: University of Washington.

94. Wuyts, W., Schmale, G.A., Chansky, H.A., and Raskind, W.H. (1993). Hereditary multiple osteochondromas. In: *GeneReviews*® (ed. M.P. Adam, H.H. Ardinger, R.A. Pagon, et al.). Seattle, WA: University of Washington.

95. Klein, R.J., Zeiss, C., Chew, E.Y. et al. (2005). Complement factor H polymorphism in age-related macular degeneration. *Science* 308: 385–389.

96. Tam, V., Patel, N., Turcotte, M. et al. (2019). Benefits and limitations of genome-wide association studies. *Nat. Rev. Genet.* 20: 467–484.

97. Sloan-Heggen, C.M., Bierer, A.O., Shearer, A.E. et al. (2016). Comprehensive genetic testing in the clinical evaluation of 1119 patients with hearing loss. *Hum. Genet.* 135: 441–450.

98. Shearer, A.E., Hildebrand, M.S., and Smith, R.J.H. (1993). Hereditary hearing loss and deafness overview. In: *GeneReviews®* (ed. M.P. Adam, H.H. Ardinger, R.A. Pagon, et al.). Seattle, WA: University of Washington.

99. Prior, T.W., Leach, M.E., and Finanger, E. (1993). Spinal muscular atrophy. In: *GeneReviews®* (ed. M.P. Adam, H.H. Ardinger, R.A. Pagon, et al.). Seattle, WA: University of Washington.

100. Gordon, L.B., Brown, W.T., and Collins, F.S. (1993). Hutchinson-Gilford progeria syndrome. In: *GeneReviews®* (ed. M.P. Adam, H.H. Ardinger, R.A. Pagon, et al.). Seattle, WA: University of Washington.

101. Merideth, M.A., Gordon, L.B., Clauss, S. et al. (2008). Phenotype and course of Hutchinson-Gilford progeria syndrome. *N. Engl. J. Med.* 358: 592–604.

102. Aubourg, P. and Wanders, R. (2013). Peroxisomal disorders. *Handb. Clin. Neurol.* 113: 1593–1609.

103. Steinberg, S.J., Raymond, G.V., Braverman, N.E., and Moser, A.B. (1993). Zellweger spectrum disorder. In: *GeneReviews®* (ed. M.P. Adam, H.H. Ardinger, R.A. Pagon, et al.). Seattle, WA: University of Washington.

104. Seemanova, E., Jarolim, P., Seeman, P. et al. (2007). Cancer risk of heterozygotes with the NBN founder mutation. *J. Natl. Cancer Inst.* 99: 1875–1880.

105. Varon, R., Demuth, I., and Chrzanowska, K.H. (1993). Nijmegen breakage syndrome. In: *GeneReviews®* (ed. M.P. Adam, H.H. Ardinger, R.A. Pagon, et al.). Seattle, WA: University of Washington.

106. Rinaldo, P., Cowan, T.M., and Matern, D. (2008). Acylcarnitine profile analysis. *Genet. Med.* 10: 151–156.

107. Boyce, A.M., Florenzano, P., de Castro, L.F., and Collins, M.T. (1993). Fibrous dysplasia/McCune-Albright syndrome. In: *GeneReviews®* (ed. M.P. Adam, H.H. Ardinger, R.A. Pagon, et al.). Seattle, WA: University of Washington.

108. Lammer, E.J., Chen, D.T., Hoar, R.M. et al. (1985). Retinoic acid embryopathy. *N. Engl. J. Med.* 313: 837–841.

109. Gorman, G.S., Chinnery, P.F., DiMauro, S. et al. (2016). Mitochondrial diseases. *Nat. Rev. Dis. Primers.* 2: 16080.

110. Chinnery, P.F. (1993). Primary mitochondrial disorders overview. In: *GeneReviews®* (ed. M.P. Adam, H.H. Ardinger, R.A. Pagon, et al.). Seattle, WA: University of Washington.

111. Brugada, R., Campuzano, O., Sarquella-Brugada, G. et al. (1993). Brugada syndrome. In: *GeneReviews®* (ed. M.P. Adam, H.H. Ardinger, R.A. Pagon, et al.). Seattle, WA: University of Washington.

112. Hosseini, S.M., Kim, R., Udupa, S. et al. (2018). Reappraisal of reported genes for sudden arrhythmic death: evidence-based evaluation of gene validity for Brugada syndrome. *Circulation* 138: 1195–1205.

113. Walsh, R., Lahrouchi, N., Tadros, R. et al. (2021). Enhancing rare variant interpretation in inherited arrhythmias through quantitative analysis of consortium disease cohorts and population controls. *Genet. Med.* 23: 47–58.

114. Visootsak, J. and Graham, J.M. Jr. (2006). Klinefelter syndrome and other sex chromosomal aneuploidies. *Orphanet J. Rare Dis.* 1: 42.

115. Nimkarn, S., Gangishetti, P.K., Yau, M., and New, M.I. (1993). 21-Hydroxylase-deficient congenital adrenal hyperplasia. In: *GeneReviews®* (ed. M.P. Adam, H.H. Ardinger, R.A. Pagon, et al.). Seattle, WA: University of Washington.

Chapter 4

116. El-Maouche, D., Arlt, W., and Merke, D.P. (2017). Congenital adrenal hyperplasia. *Lancet* 390: 2194–2210.
117. Fruhwald, M.C., Biegel, J.A., Bourdeaut, F. et al. (2016). Atypical teratoid/rhabdoid tumors-current concepts, advances in biology, and potential future therapies. *Neuro-Oncology* 18: 764–778.
118. Nemes, K., Bens, S., Bourdeaut, F. et al. (1993). Rhabdoid tumor predisposition syndrome. In: *GeneReviews®* (ed. M.P. Adam, H.H. Ardinger, R.A. Pagon, et al.). Seattle, WA: University of Washington.
119. Johnston, J.J., Olivos-Glander, I., Killoran, C. et al. (2005). Molecular and clinical analyses of Greig cephalopolysyndactyly and Pallister-Hall syndromes: robust phenotype prediction from the type and position of GLI3 mutations. *Am. J. Hum. Genet.* 76: 609–622.
120. Biesecker, L.G. (1993). Pallister-Hall syndrome. In: *GeneReviews®* (ed. M.P. Adam, H.H. Ardinger, R.A. Pagon, et al.). Seattle, WA: University of Washington.
121. Biesecker, L.G. and Johnston, J.J. (1993). Greig cephalopolysyndactyly syndrome. In: *GeneReviews®* (ed. M.P. Adam, H.H. Ardinger, R.A. Pagon, et al.). Seattle, WA: University of Washington.
122. Malone, F.D., Ball, R.H., Nyberg, D.A. et al. (2005). First-trimester septated cystic hygroma: prevalence, natural history, and pediatric outcome. *Obstet. Gynecol.* 106: 288–294.
123. Scholl, J., Durfee, S.M., Russell, M.A. et al. (2012). First-trimester cystic hygroma: relationship of nuchal translucency thickness and outcomes. *Obstet. Gynecol.* 120: 551–559.
124. Stevenson, R.E., Allanson, J.G., Everman, D.B., and Solomon, B.D. (2016). *Human Malformations and Related Anomalies*. Oxford; New York: Oxford University Press).
125. Garavelli, L. and Mainardi, P.C. (2007). Mowat-Wilson syndrome. *Orphanet J. Rare Dis.* 2: 42.
126. Ivanovski, I., Djuric, O., Caraffi, S.G. et al. (2018). Phenotype and genotype of 87 patients with Mowat-Wilson syndrome and recommendations for care. *Genet. Med.* 20: 965–975.
127. Bockenhauer, D. and Bichet, D.G. (2015). Pathophysiology, diagnosis and management of nephrogenic diabetes insipidus. *Nat. Rev. Nephrol.* 11: 576–588.
128. Torres, R.J. and Puig, J.G. (2007). Hypoxanthine-guanine phosophoribosyltransferase (HPRT) deficiency: Lesch-Nyhan syndrome. *Orphanet J. Rare Dis.* 2: 48.
129. Jinnah, H.A. (1993). HPRT1 cisorders. In: *GeneReviews®* (ed. M.P. Adam, H.H. Ardinger, R.A. Pagon, et al.). Seattle, WA: University of Washington.
130. Weese-Mayer, D.E., Rand, C.M., Zhou, A. et al. (2017). Congenital central hypoventilation syndrome: a bedside-to-bench success story for advancing early diagnosis and treatment and improved survival and quality of life. *Pediatr. Res.* 81: 192–201.
131. Weese-Mayer, D.E., Rand, C.M., Khaytin, I. et al. (1993). Congenital central hypoventilation syndrome. In: *GeneReviews®* (ed. M.P. Adam, H.H. Ardinger, R.A. Pagon, et al.). Seattle, WA: University of Washington.
132. Basu, S., Aggarwal, P., Kakani, N., and Kumar, A. (2016). Low-dose maternal warfarin intake resulting in fetal warfarin syndrome: in search for a safe anticoagulant regimen during pregnancy. *Birth Defects Res. A Clin. Mol. Teratol.* 106: 142–147.
133. Ferreira, S., Costa, R., Malveiro, D. et al. (2018). Warfarin embryopathy: balancing maternal and fetal risks with anticoagulation therapy. *Pediatr. Neonatol.* 59: 534–535.

Chapter 4

134. Sousa, A.R., Barreira, R., and Santos, E. (2018). Low-dose warfarin maternal anticoagulation and fetal warfarin syndrome. *BMJ Case Rep.* 2018.

135. Schellenberg, G.D. and Montine, T.J. (2012). The genetics and neuropathology of Alzheimer's disease. *Acta Neuropathol.* 124: 305–323.

136. Cacace, R., Sleegers, K., and Van Broeckhoven, C. (2016). Molecular genetics of early-onset Alzheimer's disease revisited. *Alzheimers Dement.* 12: 733–748.

137. Bird, T.D. (1993). Alzheimer disease overview. In: *GeneReviews®* (ed. M.P. Adam, H.H. Ardinger, R.A. Pagon, et al.). Seattle, WA: University of Washington.

138. Zhang, B., Dearing, L., and Amos, J. (2004). DNA-based carrier screening in the Ashkenazi Jewish population. *Expert. Rev. Mol. Diagn.* 4: 377–392.

139. Rose, N.C. and Wick, M. (2018). Carrier screening for single gene disorders. *Semin. Fetal Neonatal Med.* 23: 78–84.

140. King, J.R. and Klugman, S. (2018). Ethnicity-based carrier screening. *Obstet. Gynecol. Clin. N. Am.* 45: 83–101.

141. Rosenberg, A.Z. and Kopp, J.B. (2017). Focal segmental glomerulosclerosis. *Clin. J. Am. Soc. Nephrol.* 12: 502–517.

142. Freedman, B.I., Limou, S., Ma, L., and Kopp, J.B. (2018). APOL1-associated nephropathy: a key contributor to racial disparities in CKD. *Am. J. Kidney Dis.* 72: S8–S16.

143. Kopp, J.B. and Winkler, C.A. (2018). Genetics, genomics, and precision medicine in end-stage kidney disease. *Semin. Nephrol.* 38: 317–324.

144. Adam, M.P., Banka, S., Bjornsson, H.T. et al. (2019). Kabuki syndrome: international consensus diagnostic criteria. *J. Med. Genet.* 56: 89–95.

145. Adam, M.P., Hudgins, L., and Hannibal, M. (1993). Kabuki syndrome. In: *GeneReviews®* (ed. M.P. Adam, H.H. Ardinger, R.A. Pagon, et al.). Seattle, WA: University of Washington.

146. Bianchi, D.W. and Wilkins-Haug, L. (2014). Integration of noninvasive DNA testing for aneuploidy into prenatal care: what has happened since the rubber met the road? *Clin. Chem.* 60: 78–87.

147. (2016). Practice bulletin no. 163: screening for fetal aneuploidy. *Obstet. Gynecol.* 127: e123–e137.

148. Taylor-Phillips, S., Freeman, K., Geppert, J. et al. (2016). Accuracy of non-invasive prenatal testing using cell-free DNA for detection of Down, Edwards and Patau syndromes: a systematic review and meta-analysis. *BMJ Open* 6: e010002.

149. Green, R.C., Berg, J.S., Grody, W.W. et al. (2013). ACMG recommendations for reporting of incidental findings in clinical exome and genome sequencing. *Genet. Med.* 15: 565–574.

150. Kalia, S.S., Adelman, K., Bale, S.J. et al. (2017). Recommendations for reporting of secondary findings in clinical exome and genome sequencing, 2016 update (ACMG SF v2.0): a policy statement of the American College of Medical Genetics and Genomics. *Genet. Med.* 19: 249–255.

151. Miller, D.T., Lee, K., Chung, W.K. et al. (2021). ACMG SF v3.0 list for reporting of secondary findings in clinical exome and genome sequencing: a policy statement of the American College of Medical Genetics and Genomics (ACMG). *Genet. Med.* 23: 1381–1390.

152. Chinsky, J.M., Singh, R., Ficicioglu, C. et al. (2017). Diagnosis and treatment of tyrosinemia type I: a US and Canadian consensus group review and recommendations. *Genet. Med.* 19.

153. Lane, E.B. and McLean, W.H. (2004). Keratins and skin disorders. *J. Pathol.* 204: 355–366.

154. Irvine, A.D. (2005). Inherited defects in keratins. *Clin. Dermatol.* 23: 6–14.

155. Jacob, J.T., Coulombe, P.A., Kwan, R., and Omary, M.B. (2018). Types I and II keratin intermediate filaments. *Cold Spring Harb. Perspect. Biol.* 10.

156. Eisenkraft, A., Pode-Shakked, B., Goldstein, N. et al. (2015). Clinical variability in a family with an ectodermal dysplasia syndrome and a nonsense mutation in the TP63 gene. *Fetal Pediatr. Pathol.* 34: 400–406.

157. Wenger, T., Li, D., Harr, M.H. et al. (2018). Expanding the phenotypic spectrum of TP63-related disorders including the first set of monozygotic twins. *Am. J. Med. Genet. A* 176: 75–81.

158. Sutton, V.R. and van Bokhoven, H. (1993). TP63-related disorders. In: *GeneReviews®* (ed. M.P. Adam, H.H. Ardinger, R.A. Pagon, et al.). Seattle, WA: University of Washington.

159. Cardoso, L., Stevenson, M., and Thakker, R.V. (2017). Molecular genetics of syndromic and non-syndromic forms of parathyroid carcinoma. *Hum. Mutat.* 38: 1621–1648.

160. van der Tuin, K., Tops, C.M.J., Adank, M.A. et al. (2017). CDC73-related disorders: clinical manifestations and case detection in primary hyperparathyroidism. *J. Clin. Endocrinol. Metab.* 102: 4534–4540.

161. Hyde, S.M., Rich, T.A., Waguespack, S.G. et al. (1993). CDC73-related disorders. In: *GeneReviews®* (ed. M.P. Adam, H.H. Ardinger, R.A. Pagon, et al.). Seattle, WA: University of Washington.

162. Raymond, V.M., Gray, S.W., Roychowdhury, S. et al. (2016). Germline findings in tumor-only sequencing: points to consider for clinicians and laboratories. *J. Natl. Cancer Inst.* 108.

163. Uzilov, A.V., Ding, W., Fink, M.Y. et al. (2016). Development and clinical application of an integrative genomic approach to personalized cancer therapy. *Genome Med.* 8: 62.

164. Li, M.M., Datto, M., Duncavage, E.J. et al. (2017). Standards and guidelines for the interpretation and reporting of sequence variants in cancer: a joint consensus recommendation of the Association for Molecular Pathology, American Society of Clinical Oncology, and College of American Pathologists. *J. Mol. Diagn.* 19: 4–23.

165. Flanigan, K.M. (2014). Duchenne and Becker muscular dystrophies. *Neurol. Clin.* 32: 671–688, viii.

166. Aartsma-Rus, A., Ginjaar, I.B., and Bushby, K. (2016). The importance of genetic diagnosis for Duchenne muscular dystrophy. *J. Med. Genet.* 53: 145–151.

167. Darras, B.T., Urion, D.K., and Ghosh, P.S. (1993). Dystrophinopathies. In: *GeneReviews®* (ed. M.P. Adam, H.H. Ardinger, R.A. Pagon, et al.). Seattle, WA: University of Washington.

168. Ewing, C.M., Ray, A.M., Lange, E.M. et al. (2012). Germline mutations in HOXB13 and prostate-cancer risk. *N. Engl. J. Med.* 366: 141–149.

169. Dias, A., Kote-Jarai, Z., Mikropoulos, C., and Eeles, R. (2018). Prostate cancer germline variations and implications for screening and treatment. *Cold Spring Harb. Perspect. Med.* 8.

170. Giri, V.N., Knudsen, K.E., Kelly, W.K. et al. (2018). Role of genetic testing for inherited prostate cancer risk: Philadelphia Prostate Cancer Consensus Conference 2017. *J. Clin. Oncol.* 36: 414–424.

Chapter 4

171. Zhen, J.T., Syed, J., Nguyen, K.A. et al. (2018). Genetic testing for hereditary prostate cancer: current status and limitations. *Cancer* 124: 3105–3117.

172. Wang, B., Rudnick, S., Cengia, B., and Bonkovsky, H.L. (2019). Acute hepatic porphyrias: review and recent progress. *Hepatol. Commun.* 3: 193–206.

173. Bonkovsky, H.L., Dixon, N., and Rudnick, S. (2019). Pathogenesis and clinical features of the acute hepatic porphyrias (AHPs). *Mol. Genet. Metab.* 128: 213–218.

174. Whatley, S.D. and Badminton, M.N. (1993). Acute intermittent porphyria. In: *GeneReviews®* (ed. M.P. Adam, H.H. Ardinger, R.A. Pagon, et al.). Seattle, WA: University of Washington.

175. Burton, B.K. (1998). Inborn errors of metabolism in infancy: a guide to diagnosis. *Pediatrics* 102: E69.

176. Levy, P.A. (2009). Inborn errors of metabolism: part 1: overview. *Pediatr. Rev.* 30: 131–137; quiz 137–138.

177. Larsen Haidle, J. and Howe, J.R. (1993). Juvenile polyposis syndrome. In: *GeneReviews®* (ed. M.P. Adam, H.H. Ardinger, R.A. Pagon, et al.). Seattle, WA: University of Washington.

178. Boycott, K.M., Vanstone, M.R., Bulman, D.E., and MacKenzie, A.E. (2013). Rare-disease genetics in the era of next-generation sequencing: discovery to translation. *Nat. Rev. Genet.* 14: 681–691.

179. Clark, M.M., Hildreth, A., Batalov, S. et al. (2019). Diagnosis of genetic diseases in seriously ill children by rapid whole-genome sequencing and automated phenotyping and interpretation. *Sci. Transl. Med.* 11: eaat6177.

180. Short, P.J., McRae, J.F., Gallone, G. et al. (2018). De novo mutations in regulatory elements in neurodevelopmental disorders. *Nature* 555: 611–616.

181. Bamshad, M.J., Nickerson, D.A., and Chong, J.X. (2019). Mendelian gene discovery: fast and furious with no end in sight. *Am. J. Hum. Genet.* 105: 448–455.

182. Wells, A., Heckerman, D., Torkamani, A. et al. (2019). Ranking of non-coding pathogenic variants and putative essential regions of the human genome. *Nat. Commun.* 10: 5241.

183. Lunati, A., Lesage, S., and Brice, A. (2018). The genetic landscape of Parkinson's disease. *Rev. Neurol.* 174: 628–643.

184. Marsh, S.G., Albert, E.D., Bodmer, W.F. et al. (2005). Nomenclature for factors of the HLA system, 2004. *Hum. Immunol.* 66: 571–636.

185. Dendrou, C.A., Petersen, J., Rossjohn, J., and Fugger, L. (2018). HLA variation and disease. *Nat. Rev. Immunol.* 18: 325–339.

186. Eber, S.W., Gonzalez, J.M., Lux, M.L. et al. (1996). Ankyrin-1 mutations are a major cause of dominant and recessive hereditary spherocytosis. *Nat. Genet.* 13: 214–218.

187. Tole, S., Dhir, P., Pugi, J. et al. (2020). Genotype-phenotype correlation in children with hereditary spherocytosis. *Br. J. Haematol.* 191: 486–496.

188. Eagles, N., Sebire, N.J., Short, D. et al. (2015). Risk of recurrent molar pregnancies following complete and partial hydatidiform moles. *Hum. Reprod.* 30: 2055–2063.

189. Hui, P., Buza, N., Murphy, K.M., and Ronnett, B.M. (2017). Hydatidiform moles: genetic basis and precision diagnosis. *Annu. Rev. Pathol.* 12: 449–485.

190. Nguyen, N.M.P., Khawajkie, Y., Mechtouf, N. et al. (2018). The genetics of recurrent hydatidiform moles: new insights and lessons from a comprehensive analysis of 113 patients. *Mod. Pathol.* 31: 1116–1130.

Chapter 4

191. Nagy, R., Sweet, K., and Eng, C. (2004). Highly penetrant hereditary cancer syndromes. *Oncogene* 23: 6445–6470.
192. Yehia, L. and Eng, C. (1993). PTEN hamartoma tumor syndrome. In: *GeneReviews®* (ed. M.P. Adam, H.H. Ardinger, R.A. Pagon, et al.). Seattle, WA: University of Washington.
193. Kwon, J.M., Matern, D., Kurtzberg, J. et al. (2018). Consensus guidelines for newborn screening, diagnosis and treatment of infantile Krabbe disease. *Orphanet J. Rare Dis.* 13: 30.
194. Orsini, J.J., Escolar, M.L., Wasserstein, M.P., and Caggana, M. (1993). Krabbe disease. In: *GeneReviews®* (ed. M.P. Adam, H.H. Ardinger, R.A. Pagon, et al.). Seattle, WA: University of Washington.
195. Komatsuzaki, S., Zielonka, M., Mountford, W.K. et al. (2019). Clinical characteristics of 248 patients with Krabbe disease: quantitative natural history modeling based on published cases. *Genet. Med.* 21: 2208–2215.
196. Lachman, R.S., Tiller, G.E., Graham, J.M. Jr., and Rimoin, D.L. (1992). Collagen, genes and the skeletal dysplasias on the edge of a new era: a review and update. *Eur. J. Radiol.* 14: 1–10.
197. Besio, R., Chow, C.W., Tonelli, F. et al. (2019). Bone biology: insights from osteogenesis imperfecta and related rare fragility syndromes. *FEBS J.* 286: 3033–3056.
198. Marini, J.C. and Dang Do, A.N. (2000). Osteogenesis imperfecta. In: *Endotext [Internet]* (ed. K.R. Feingold, B. Anawalt, A. Boyce, et al.). South Dartmouth, MA: MDText.com, Inc.
199. Feuchtbaum, L., Carter, J., Dowray, S. et al. (2012). Birth prevalence of disorders detectable through newborn screening by race/ethnicity. *Genet. Med.* 14: 937–945.
200. Fridovich-Keil, J.L., Gambello, M.J., Singh, R.H., and Sharer, J.D. (1993). Duarte variant galactosemia. In: *GeneReviews®* (ed. M.P. Adam, H.H. Ardinger, R.A. Pagon, et al.). Seattle, WA: University of Washington.
201. Wilkin, D.J., Szabo, J.K., Cameron, R. et al. (1998). Mutations in fibroblast growth-factor receptor 3 in sporadic cases of achondroplasia occur exclusively on the paternally derived chromosome. *Am. J. Hum. Genet.* 63: 711–716.
202. Acuna-Hidalgo, R., Veltman, J.A., and Hoischen, A. (2016). New insights into the generation and role of de novo mutations in health and disease. *Genome Biol.* 17: 241.
203. Dietz, H. (1993). Marfan syndrome. In: *GeneReviews®* (ed. M.P. Adam, H.H. Ardinger, R.A. Pagon, et al.). Seattle, WA: University of Washington.
204. Friedman, J.M. (1993). Neurofibromatosis 1. In: *GeneReviews®* (ed. M.P. Adam, H.H. Ardinger, R.A. Pagon, et al.). Seattle, WA: University of Washington.
205. Legare, J.M. (1993). Achondroplasia. In: *GeneReviews®* (ed. M.P. Adam, H.H. Ardinger, R.A. Pagon, et al.). Seattle, WA: University of Washington.
206. Northrup, H., Koenig, M.K., Pearson, D.A., and Au, K.S. (1993). Tuberous sclerosis complex. In: *GeneReviews®* (ed. M.P. Adam, H.H. Ardinger, R.A. Pagon, et al.). Seattle, WA: University of Washington.
207. Gripp, K.W., Schill, L., Schoyer, L. et al. (2020). The sixth international RASopathies symposium: precision medicine-From promise to practice. *Am. J. Med. Genet. A* 182: 597–606.
208. Gross, A.M., Frone, M., Gripp, K.W. et al. (2020). Advancing RAS/RASopathy therapies: An NCI-sponsored intramural and extramural collaboration for the study of RASopathies. *Am. J. Med. Genet. A* 182: 866–876.

Chapter 4

209. Jerome, L.A. and Papaioannou, V.E. (2001). DiGeorge syndrome phenotype in mice mutant for the T-box gene, Tbx1. *Nat. Genet.* 27: 286–291.
210. Yagi, H., Furutani, Y., Hamada, H. et al. (2003). Role of TBX1 in human del22q11.2 syndrome. *Lancet* 362: 1366–1373.
211. Paylor, R., Glaser, B., Mupo, A. et al. (2006). Tbx1 haploinsufficiency is linked to behavioral disorders in mice and humans: implications for 22q11 deletion syndrome. *Proc. Natl Acad. Sci. USA* 103: 7729–7734.

212. Zweier, C., Sticht, H., Aydin-Yaylagul, I. et al. (2007). Human TBX1 missense mutations cause gain of function resulting in the same phenotype as 22q11.2 deletions. *Am. J. Hum. Genet.* 80: 510–517.
213. Lindhurst, M.J., Sapp, J.C., Teer, J.K. et al. (2011). A mosaic activating mutation in AKT1 associated with the Proteus syndrome. *N. Engl. J. Med.* 365: 611–619.
214. Levy-Lahad, E. and King, M.C. (2020). Hiding in plain sight – somatic mutation in human disease. *N. Engl. J. Med.* 383: 2680–2682.
215. Lawrence, R., Brown, J.R., Lorey, F. et al. (2014). Glycan-based biomarkers for mucopolysaccharidoses. *Mol. Genet. Metab.* 111: 73–83.
216. Kubaski, F., de Oliveira Poswar, F., Michelin-Tirelli, K. et al. (2020). Diagnosis of mucopolysaccharidoses. *Diagnostics* 10: 172.
217. National Human Genome Research Institute: Elements of Morphology: Human Malformation Terminology. https://elementsofmorphology.nih.gov/ (accessed 26 July 21).
218. Ranke, M.B. and Saenger, P. (2001). Turner's syndrome. *Lancet* 358: 309–314.
219. Kruszka, P. and Silberbach, M. (2019). The state of Turner syndrome science: are we on the threshold of discovery? *Am. J. Med. Genet. C Semin. Med. Genet.* 181: 4–6.
220. San Roman, A.K. and Page, D.C. (2019). A strategic research alliance: Turner syndrome and sex differences. *Am. J. Med. Genet. C Semin. Med. Genet.* 181: 59–67.
221. Zhuang, Z., Park, W.S., Pack, S. et al. (1998). Trisomy 7-harbouring non-random duplication of the mutant MET allele in hereditary papillary renal carcinomas. *Nat. Genet.* 20: 66–69.
222. Yang, X.J., Tan, M.H., Kim, H.L. et al. (2005). A molecular classification of papillary renal cell carcinoma. *Cancer Res.* 65: 5628–5637.
223. Dizman, N., Philip, E.J., and Pal, S.K. (2020). Genomic profiling in renal cell carcinoma. *Nat. Rev. Nephrol.* 16: 435–451.
224. Hernandez-Martin, A., Gonzalez-Sarmiento, R., and De Unamuno, P. (1999). X-linked ichthyosis: an update. *Br. J. Dermatol.* 141: 617–627.
225. Fischer, J. and Bourrat, E. (2020). Genetics of Inherited Ichthyoses and Related Diseases. *Acta Derm. Venereol.* 100: adv00096.

Management of Genetic Conditions and Therapeutics

5

5.1. Individuals with what type of mitochondrial disorder are most likely to benefit from treatment with riboflavin?
   A. Complexes I and II
   B. Complex III
   C. Complex IV
   D. Kearns-Sayre syndrome

5.2. In people with Loeys-Dietz syndrome, which of the following is a relatively common complication that requires monitoring and potential interventions?
   A. Arterial aneurysms
   B. Colorectal cancer
   C. Ectopia lentis
   D. Immunodeficiency

5.3. A person has Familial Mediterranean fever (with pathogenic variants identified in *MEFV*). What treatment is most likely to be beneficial?
   A. Amoxicillin
   B. Colchicine
   C. Colectomy
   D. Levetiracetam

5.4. A pregnant woman has high phenylalanine due to poorly controlled Phenylketonuria. Due to this, she may be at elevated risk to have a child with what type of congenital anomaly?
   A. Cardiac malformations
   B. Epidermolysis bullosa
   C. Macrosomia
   D. Polydactyly

5.5. Which class of medications is most associated with causing clinical manifestations of Malignant hyperthermia?
   A. Anesthetics
   B. Antibiotics
   C. Antiemetics
   D. Antiepileptics

5.6. People with Xeroderma pigmentosum are particularly sensitive to the effects of what?
   A. Fungal infections
   B. Hypoglycemia
   C. Pain medication
   D. Sunlight

5.7. What treatment may be helpful for patients with conditions due to pathogenic variants in *GAMT* or *GATM*?
   A. Amoxicillin
   B. Hormone replacement
   C. Liver transplant
   D. Oral creatine

5.8. A pregnant patient has signs of a possible connective tissue disorder. Which condition/syndrome includes the highest risk of uterine rupture?
   A. Diastrophic dysplasia
   B. Orofaciodigital syndrome
   C. Stickler syndrome
   D. Vascular Ehlers-Danlos syndrome

Medical Genetics and Genomics: Questions for Board Review, First Edition. Benjamin D. Solomon.
© 2023 John Wiley & Sons Ltd. Published 2023 by John Wiley & Sons Ltd.

5.9. An individual has a pathogenic variant in the *FH* gene. In addition to leiomyomatosis (smooth muscle tumors), the person would most likely require management for what main type of cancer?
A. Lung
B. Melanoma
C. Renal
D. Thyroid

5.10. For which condition is there an FDA-approved gene therapy available?
A. Lesch-Nyhan syndrome
B. Macular dystrophy
C. Phenylketonuria
D. Spinal muscular atrophy

5.11. Untreated, which of the following conditions typically results in rickets, short stature, photophobia, and renal failure?
A. Acromegaly
B. Cystinosis
C. Hermansky-Pudlak syndrome
D. Marfan syndrome

5.12. Which gene/protein family encodes enzymes that are especially important for the metabolism of many medications?
A. Cytochrome P450 (CYP)
B. Homeobox
C. Olfactory receptor
D. WNT

5.13. Which of the following is the most common trigger of hemolysis in patients with Glucose-6-phosphate dehydrogenase (G6PD) deficiency?
A. Fava beans
B. Infections
C. NSAIDs
D. Sulfa drugs

5.14. For children with PTEN hamartoma tumor syndrome (PHTS), what yearly surveillance has been recommended?
A. Echocardiogram
B. Electroencephalogram (EEG)
C. Thyroid ultrasound
D. Whole-body MRI

5.15. Which of the following is the most common sequelae of untreated congenital hypothyroidism?
A. Cancer
B. Hyperthyroidism
C. Immunodeficiency
D. Intellectual disability

5.16. Brown-Vialetto-Van Laere and Fazio-Londe syndromes involve deficient transport of what substance (and, therefore, related treatment is based on supplements of this substance)?
A. Copper
B. Lead
C. Riboflavin
D. Zinc

5.17. A patient has Thrombocytopenia absent radius (TAR) syndrome. What treatment would be most likely to be required?
A. Biotin supplementation
B. Kidney transplant
C. Plasmapharesis
D. Platelet transfusion

5.18. An infant has been diagnosed with congenital asplenia. What management consideration or next step would likely be most important?
A. EEG
B. Enzyme replacement
C. Liver transplant
D. Pneumococcal vaccine

5.19. A child weaning from breastfeeding is frequently vomiting, has signs of abdominal pain, and is demonstrating failure to thrive. The child is eventually found to have compound heterozygous variants in *ALDOB*. Limitation of exposure to which of the following would be recommended?

A. Any protein
B. Fructose/sucrose/sorbitol
C. Galactose/glucose
D. Penicillin/vancomycin

5.20. An acutely ill patient with a known urea cycle disorder comes to the emergency department. Which of the following lab tests would likely be the most helpful to guide immediate care?

A. Ammonia
B. CRP and ESR
C. Homocysteine
D. Karyotype

5.21. An infant is found to have Biotinidase deficiency by newborn screening. For this patient, administration of oral biotin therapy is usually necessary for how long or for what time period?

A. After adolescence
B. Lifelong
C. Only during "attacks"
D. Only in infancy

5.22. In a person with Oculocutaneous albinism, being followed by what type of medical specialist regularly is often indicated?

A. Anesthesiologist
B. Gastroenterologist
C. Nephrologist
D. Ophthalmologist

5.23. In a child who has Down syndrome, what test is recommended to be performed annually starting at about one year of age (and more often in the first year of life)?

A. Echocardiogram
B. Full CBC with differential
C. Liver function testing
D. TSH

5.24. For which of the following conditions/diseases is enzyme replacement therapy NOT currently clinically available?

A. ADA-SCID
B. Gaucher disease
C. Pompe disease
D. Tay-Sachs disease

5.25. Due to family history, a child has been identified as affected by Familial adenomatous polyposis (FAP). Based on current recommendations, at approximately what age should colorectal screening begin?

A. 5 years
B. 10 years
C. 25 years
D. 45 years

5.26. Due to physical examination and family history findings suggestive of a genetic condition, a person has been found to have a pathogenic variant in *FBN1*. Based on this, what medical treatment would most likely be indicated (though this would only be indicated for some conditions related to this gene)?

A. Anakinra
B. Beta blocker
C. Carnitine
D. Digoxin

5.27. In a patient with certain types of cancer, identification of a germline pathogenic variant in *BRCA1* or *BRCA2* might lead to consideration of therapy with what type of agent?

A. AAV9-based gene therapy
B. Nitrosourea
C. PARP inhibitor
D. PD-1 inhibitor

5.28. A two-year-old girl has been diagnosed with Rett syndrome. In addition to supportive and other care, what type of surveillance is recommended based on this diagnosis?

A. Colonoscopy

B. Electrocardiogram

C. LH and FSH levels

D. Melanoma screening

5.29. Tisagenlecleucel was the first form of gene therapy to be FDA-approved for use in the United States. This treatment, for a form of acute lymphoblastic leukemia, is considered what type of therapy?

A. CAR-T

B. CRISPR

C. Enzyme replacement

D. RNA interference

5.30. A patient with neonatal-onset epilepsy has been found to have biallelic pathogenic variants in the gene *ALDH7A1*. What treatment might be effective based on this genetic information?

A. Allopurinol

B. Colchicine

C. Levodopa

D. Pyridoxine

Answers

5.1. A	5.9. C	2.17. D	2.25. B
5.2. A	5.10. D	2.18. D	2.26. B
5.3. B	2.11. B	2.19. B	2.27. C
5.4. A	2.12. A	2.20. A	2.28. B
5.5. A	2.13. B	2.21. B	2.29. A
5.6. D	2.14. C	2.22. D	5.30. D
5.7. D	2.15. D	2.23. D	
5.8. D	2.16. C	2.24. D	

Commentary

5.1. Complexes I and II

Mitochondrial disorders can be caused by pathogenic variants affecting the mitochondrial DNA or nuclear DNA. There can be a wide range of manifestations and severity. The management of some mitochondrial disorders is supportive, but patients with certain types of mitochondrial disease can benefit from specific treatment. Riboflavin may be beneficial for patients with mitochondrial complex I and/or complex II deficiency.

Reference(s): Parikh et al. [1]; Chinnery [2].

5.2. Arterial aneurysms

Loeys-Dietz syndrome (LDS) involves cerebral, thoracic, and abdominal arterial aneurysms/dissections, skeletal manifestations (including pectus anomalies, scoliosis, joint laxity or contracture, arachnodactyly, talipes equinovarus, and cervical spine anomalies), and craniofacial and cutaneous findings. LDS can be caused by heterozygous pathogenic variants in several different genes, and there are some genotype–phenotype correlations depending on the gene involved. Arterial aneurysms are typically aggressive, and surveillance and management are important for the care of affected individuals.

Reference(s): Verstraeten et al. [3]; Loeys and Dietz [4].

5.3. Colchicine

Familial Mediterranean fever (FMF) is an autoinflammatory condition caused by pathogenic variants in the gene *MEFV*. Clinical features of FMF include recurrent episodes of fever, skin eruption, and abdominal, chest, and joint pain, as well as laboratory findings of elevated ESR, leukocytosis, and elevated serum fibrinogen. Management is multifaceted, including supportive care of acute episodes and medical management with colchicine in order to prevent inflammatory attacks and amyloid deposition. The decision to use colchicine for treatment in an individual is based on information such as the specific genetic changes identified as well as the person's clinical features.

Reference(s): Ozen et al. [5]; Shohat [6].

5.4. Cardiac malformations

Mothers with Phenylketonuria (PKU) due to phenylalanine hydroxylase (PAH) deficiency who have a consistently high concentration of phenylalanine during early gestation have an ~10% risk of having children with cardiac malformations. Additional findings for which these children are at elevated risk include microcephaly and neurocognitive dysfunction, and intrauterine growth restriction. Other anomalies have also been described in the children of mothers with PKU. To minimize these risks, it is recommended that women with PAH deficiency follow a phenylalanine-restricted diet prior to and during pregnancy and have ongoing dietary and biochemical monitoring.

Reference(s): Singh et al. [7]; Regier and Greene [8].

5.5. Anesthetics

Malignant hyperthermia (MH) is a life-threatening condition that involves abnormal metabolism of calcium by skeletal muscle. MH can be triggered by certain volatile anesthetics alone or in conjunction with a depolarizing muscle relaxant (succinylcholine). The manifestations of MH are usually first noticed in the operating room. Clinical signs, which can be fatal if untreated, include hyperthermia, tachycardia, tachypnea, acidosis, increased oxygen consumption and carbon dioxide production, muscle rigidity, hyperkalemia, and rhabdomyolysis. Early diagnosis and treatment is critical; among other management components, dantrolene sodium should be available wherever general anesthesia is used. MH can be caused by pathogenic variants in the *RYR1* or *CACNA1S* genes.

Reference(s): Rosenberg et al. [9]; Rosenberg et al. [10].

5.6. Sunlight

Xeroderma pigmentosum (XP) primarily involves marked skin and eye sun sensitivity, and includes an increased risk of skin as well as other possible neoplasms. About 25% of patients also have neurologic manifestations. XP is an autosomal recessive condition, and can be caused by biallelic pathogenic variants in multiple genes. These variants affect the ability to repair damaged DNA.

Reference(s): Kraemer and DiGiovanna [11].

5.7. Oral creatine

Cerebral creatine deficiency includes Guanidinoacetate methyltransferase (GAMT) deficiency, L-arginine : glycine amidinotransferase (AGAT) deficiency, and Creatine transporter (CRTR) deficiency. GAMT and AGAT deficiency are autosomal recessive conditions, while CRTR deficiency is X-linked. Clinical manifestations of these inborn errors of metabolism are primarily neurologic and behavioral. Diagnosis may be made via a combination of biochemical/enzymatic tests and/or molecular genetic testing of the genes involved. People with GAMT and AGAT deficiency may be treated with oral creatine monohydrate, and there is evidence that early (presymptomatic) diagnosis and treatment is beneficial. Patients with GAMT deficiency may also benefit from ornithine supplementation and arginine and/or protein restriction.

Reference(s): Clark and Cecil [12]; Mercimek-Andrews and Salomons [13].

5.8. Vascular Ehlers-Danlos syndrome

Vascular Ehlers-Danlos syndrome (vEDS), also called Ehlers-Danlos type IV, is a connective tissue disorder that involves easy bruising, translucent and thin skin, a characteristic facial appearance, and fragility of the arteries, intestines, and uterus. vEDS is caused by heterozygous pathogenic variants in *COL3A1*. In one study, life-threatening complications were described in 14.5% of deliveries: arterial dissection/rupture (9%), uterine rupture (3%), and surgical complications (3%).

Reference(s): Murray et al. [14]; Byers [15].

5.9. Renal

Hereditary leiomyomatosis and renal cell cancer (HLRCC) is due to heterozygous pathogenic variants in *FH*. Due to wider phenotypic variability in recent studies, the condition has been termed *FH* tumor predisposition syndrome. The condition frequently involves cutaneous and uterine leiomyomata (fibroids) and renal tumors, as well as other findings. About 15% of people with HLRCC have renal tumors, most of which are type 2 papillary renal cell cancer, though other types of renal neoplasms have also been described.

Reference(s): Toro et al. [16]; Wei et al. [17]; Kamihara et al. [18].

5.10. Spinal muscular atrophy

Gene therapies have been developed and tested to treat a number of genetic conditions, including a type of spinal muscular atrophy (SMA), which was FDA-approved in 2019. Gene therapy and gene editing-based treatments are being studied related to many other conditions.

Reference(s): Dunbar et al. [19]; High and Roncarlo [20].

5.11. Cystinosis

Cystinosis is an autosomal recessive lysosomal storage disorder that occurs due to pathogenic variants in the gene *CTNS*. Disease sequelae results from cystine buildup in the lysosomes. There are three forms of cystinosis: nephropathic (classic) infantile cystinosis, which is the most severe form, an intermediate form with adolescent onset, and an ocular form with corneal crystals and photophobia. Classic cystinosis, accounting for approximately 95% of cases, involves failure to thrive in infancy, renal failure, photophobia, and visual loss, as well as effects on other organs such as the thyroid.

Management can involve cystine-depleting therapy, the benefits of which are greatly increased by early diagnosis.

Reference(s): Nesterova and Gahl [21]; Nesterova and Gahl [22].

5.12. Cytochrome P450 (CYP)

The Cytochrome P450 (CYP) genes encode enzyme whose roles include the synthesis and metabolism of certain molecules and chemicals within cells, including many medications. Of dozens of functional human CYPs, about one dozen are responsible for the biotransformation of most foreign agents, including about 70–80% of all drugs in clinical use. Logically, variants in the genes that encode these enzymes can affect drug metabolism. Knowledge of a person's variants in these (as well as certain other) genes can be important in clinical practice to reduce the chance of side effects and/or non-efficacy.

Reference(s): Zanger and Schwab [23]; McCarthy and Mendelsohn [24].

5.13. Infections

Glucose-6-phosphate dehydrogenase (G6PD) deficiency is an X-linked disorder that is most commonly caused by pathogenic variants in *G6PD*. Males are more commonly and severely affected. The condition can manifest with neonatal jaundice or acute hemolytic anemia related to oxidative stress. Acute hemolytic anemia can be triggered by multiple factors, including certain foods (such as fava beans) and medications, as well as other exposures, but viral and bacterial infections are the most common inciting factors.

Reference(s): Luzzatto and Arese [25]; Nussbaum et al. [26].

5.14. Thyroid ultrasound

Heterozygous pathogenic variants (mutations) in the *PTEN* gene cause a range of phenotypic manifestations grouped together under the term "PTEN hamartoma tumor syndrome" (PHTS). According to this classification schema, PHTS includes Cowden syndrome (CS), and Bannayan-Riley-Ruvalcaba syndrome (BRRS), as well as other conditions with overlapping features. CS includes macrocephaly, skin findings such as trichilemmomas and papillomatous papules as well as increased risk for breast, endometrial, and thyroid tumors. BRRS includes macrocephaly, lipomas, pigmented macules of the glans penis, and intestinal hamartomatous polyposis. Surveillance recommendations have related to the risk of tumors, and include yearly thyroid ultrasound and skin checks in children and adults, as well as regular screening for breast and endometrial cancer in women and for colon and renal cancer in men and women.

Reference(s): Yehia and Eng [27].

5.15. Intellectual disability

Congenital hypothyroidism occurs in about 1 in 2000–4000 infants, may be due to genetic or nongenetic causes. Genetic causes, which may occur in a syndromic or nonsyndromic context, are estimated to account for up to about 20% of congenital hypothyroidism. Sequelae of congenital hypothyroidism can include intellectual disability and slow growth. Treatment with thyroid hormone, when the condition is identified early such as through newborn screening, can prevent these sequelae.

Reference(s): Grüters et al. [28]; Bodian et al. [29].

5.16. Riboflavin

Riboflavin transporter deficiency can manifest in different ways. Depending on the clinical features, the conditions are sometimes called Brown-Vialetto-Van Laere syndrome or Fazio-Londe syndrome. In general, riboflavin transporter deficiency presents in infancy or childhood (though can present later) with findings such as cranial nerve deficits, feeding difficulties, gait ataxia, and motor neuropathy. Multiple genes have been implicated in riboflavin transporter deficiency. Accurate diagnosis is important due to treatment implications such as through high-dose oral riboflavin supplementation.

Reference(s): Jaeger and Bosch [30]; Barile et al. [31]; Cali et al. [32].

5.17. Platelet transfusion

Thrombocytopenia absent radius (TAR) syndrome can be caused by the combination of a heterozygous deletion in chromosome 1q21.1 in trans with a heterozygous pathogenic variant in *RBM8A*. The condition involves bilateral absence of the radii (but the presence of thumbs) and thrombocytopenia. Among other management considerations, platelet transfusion may be required to treat thrombocytopenia.

Reference(s): Toriello [33]; Albers et al. [34]; Toriello [31].

5.18. Pneumococcal vaccine

Asplenia, or absence of the spleen, may be congenital, and may occur in an isolated or syndromic context. In the syndromic context, one important association can be with heterotaxy and related conditions, in which multiple organs may be involved in the overall disorder. In either isolated or syndromic asplenia, newly diagnosed infants (who have not already been immunized) should receive the pneumococcal vaccine. Other vaccines and anti-infectious prophylaxis are also typically warranted.

Reference(s): Stevenson et al. [35]; Salvadori et al. [36].

5.19. Fructose/sucrose/sorbitol

Hereditary fructose intolerance (HFI) is an autosomal recessive condition that can be caused by biallelic pathogenic variants in *ALDOB*. The condition often initially manifests during weaning from breastfeeding, when infants are exposed to food that contain fructose or sucrose. The manifestations can include nausea, vomiting, abdominal distress, and failure to thrive, with lab findings including hypoglycemia, lactic acidemia, hypophosphatemia, hyperuricemia, hypermagnesemia, and hyperalaninemia. Limitation of the contributing food items is an important part of management.

Reference(s): Bouteldja and Timson [37]; Demirbas et al. [38]; Gaughan et al. [39].

5.20. Ammonia

Urea cycle disorders are inborn errors of metabolism that result from pathogenic variants affecting genes encoding the enzymes involved in this biochemical process. Prompt recognition of the condition and acute management is critical, and immediate and serial measurement of plasma ammonia levels is one (of many) important parts of the care pathway for an acutely ill patient.

Reference(s): Ah Mew et al. [40]; Häberle et al. [41].

5.21. Lifelong

Biotinidase deficiency is an inborn error of metabolism caused by biallelic pathogenic variants in *BTD*. Untreated, profound biotinidase deficiency leads to neurologic manifestations (ataxia, developmental delay, hypotonia, motor limb weakness, seizures, and spastic paresis), vision problems, hearing loss, and skin abnormalities (alopecia, candidiasis, and rash). Partial biotinidase deficiency may include hair loss, hypotonia, and rash, and hair loss. Infants identified by newborn screening should remain asymptomatic with early institution and lifelong therapy with biotin.

Reference(s): Wolf [42]; Küry et al. [43]; Wolf [44].

5.22. Ophthalmologist

Oculocutaneous albinism (OCA) is a condition that involves decreased or absent melanin pigment, which affects the pigmentation of the skin, hair, and eyes. There are multiple different types of OCA, including certain syndromes that involve OCA as well as other features, and multiple known genetic causes. Among other aspects of clinical care (such as sun protection), seeing an ophthalmologist at diagnosis and for regular follow-up to monitor visual function is recommended.

Reference(s): Lewis [45]; Lewis [46].

5.23. TSH

In children with Down syndrome, specific guidelines have been devised in order to help identify and therefore manage medical issues that are more common in these individuals. Among the recommendations, annual thyroid stimulating hormone (TSH) testing to assess for hypothyroidism is recommended starting at one year of age. In the first year of life, this is recommended to be performed at birth to one month of age (this is often done as part of newborn screening), and at 6 and 12 months of age.

Reference(s): Roizen and Patterson [47]; Bull et al. [48].

5.24. Tay-Sachs disease

Enyzme replacement therapy involves medical treatment in which a patient with a condition (e.g. certain inborn errors of metabolism) involving dysfunctional or absent enzyme receives replacement enzyme. Some genetic conditions have currently available treatment through enzyme replacement therapy, including ADA-SCID (Adenosine deaminase-deficient severe combined immunodeficiency), Niemann-Pick disease type C, and Pompe disease, as well as others. There are also multiple potential enzyme replacement treatments in clinical trials. Currently, Tay-Sachs disease (due to deficiency of the hexosaminidase A enzyme) does not have clinically available enzyme replacement therapy.

Reference(s): Parenti et al. [49]; Cachon-Gonzalez et al. [50]; Flinn and Gennery [51]; Toro et al. [52].

5.25. 10 years

Familial adenomatous polyposis (FAP) results from heterozygous pathogenic variants in *APC*. Among other features, FAP involves thousands of adenomatous colonic polyps and a high risk of colon cancer; polyps can also affect other parts of the gastrointestinal tract. In people with FAP, it has been recommended that colorectal screening be initiated starting at 10–12 years of age. Additional surveillance and management considerations are also important. There are also other, related conditions involving the *APC* gene, and there are specific recommendations for these conditions. For example, for people with a condition known as attenuated FAP, colorectal screening is recommended to begin later than for people with FAP.

Reference(s): Jasperson et al. [53]; NCCN [54].

5.26. Beta blocker

Marfan syndrome, as well as multiple other conditions, can be caused by pathogenic variants in *FBN1*. Marfan syndrome affects multiple organ systems, including the eyes, musculoskeletal system, and cardiovascular system. Among other management considerations, medical management of cardiovascular sequelae with beta blockers and/or angiotensin receptor blockers is often used to help reduce hemodynamic stress on the aortic wall.

Reference(s): Dietz [55]; Milewicz et al. [56].

5.27. PARP inhibitor

Pathogenic variants in *BRCA1* or *BRCA2* can be involved in an increased risk of multiple types of cancer, including breast cancer (in both males and females), ovarian cancer, and prostate cancer. The presence of variants in specific genes may help drive the selection of therapies as well as the overall management strategy for many types of cancer; this may be true of variants found in the tumors (often called "somatic variants" in this context) or germline variants. Clinical trials have shown efficacy of PARP (poly-ADP ribose polymerase) inhibitors (e.g. olaparib, niraparib, and rucaparib) for individuals with certain cancer types related to germline pathogenic variants in *BRCA1* or *BRCA2*, and drugs in this class have been approved in certain scenarios.

Reference(s): King et al. [57]; Litton et al. [58]; Cheng et al. [59]; Mohyuddin et al. [60].

5.28. Electrocardiogram

Classic Rett syndrome is described in females who have apparently normal cognitive development until about 18 months of age, followed by developmental stagnation, regression, and then long-term stability. The condition is now considered a spectrum of disease that can arise from pathogenic variants affecting *MECP2*; similar presentations can involve other genes. One complication of Rett syndrome can include a prolonged corrected QT (QTc) interval, and surveillance via electrocardiogram has been recommended due to this finding, with cardiac follow-up if a prolonged QTc is detected.

Reference(s): Ellaway et al. [61]; Crosson et al. [62]; Kaur et al. [63].

5.29. CAR-T

Tisagenlecleucel, a form of gene therapy to treat B-cell acute lymphoblastic leukemia (ALL), was approved by the FDA in 2017. In this approach, T cells are removed from the patient, and are genetically modified to create a chimeric receptor on the surface of the T cells. That is, a gene to make a chimeric antigen receptor (CAR) is added to the T cells – this is why this type of therapy is sometimes called "CAR-T" therapy. After this is done in the laboratory, the modified cells are transferred back to the patient. Since the approval of tisagenlecleucel, gene therapies to treat other conditions have also been approved in the United States.

Reference(s): Maude et al. [64]; Maude et al. [65].

5.30. Pyridoxine

There are many different genetic causes of seizure disorders. Sometimes, knowing the molecular genetic cause can be important to determine the optimal treatment. Individuals with biallelic pathogenic variants in *ALDH7A1* may have Pyridoxine-responsive epilepsy. The condition manifests with neonatal-onset seizures, and is unresponsive to standard antiepileptic drugs, but, as the name implies, will respond to treatment with pyridoxine. Adjunctive therapy (lysine reduction therapies) has also been recommended for patients with this condition.

Reference(s): Mills et al. [66]; Olson et al. [67]; Coughlin et al. [68].

References

1. Parikh, S., Saneto, R., Falk, M.J. et al. (2009). A modern approach to the treatment of mitochondrial disease. *Curr. Treat. Options Neurol.* 11: 414–430.
2. Chinnery, P.F. (1993). Primary mitochondrial disorders overview. In: *GeneReviews®* (ed. M.P. Adam, H.H. Ardinger, R.A. Pagon, et al.). Seattle, WA: University of Washington.
3. Verstraeten, A., Alaerts, M., Van Laer, L., and Loeys, B. (2016). Marfan syndrome and related disorders: 25 years of gene discovery. *Hum. Mutat.* 37: 524–531.
4. Loeys, B.L. and Dietz, H.C. (1993). Loeys-Dietz syndrome. In: *GeneReviews®* (ed. M.P. Adam, H.H. Ardinger, R.A. Pagon, et al.). Seattle, WA: University of Washington.
5. Ozen, S., Demirkaya, E., Erer, B. et al. (2016). EULAR recommendations for the management of familial Mediterranean fever. *Ann. Rheum. Dis.* 75: 644–651.
6. Shohat, M. (1993). Familial mediterranean fever. In: *GeneReviews®* (ed. M.P. Adam, H.H. Ardinger, R.A. Pagon, et al.). Seattle, WA: University of Washington.
7. Singh, R.H., Cunningham, A.C., Mofidi, S. et al. (2016). Updated, web-based nutrition management guideline for PKU: an evidence and consensus based approach. *Mol. Genet. Metab.* 118: 72–83.
8. Regier, D.S. and Greene, C.L. (1993). Phenylalanine hydroxylase deficiency. In: *GeneReviews®* (ed. M.P. Adam, H.H. Ardinger, R.A. Pagon, et al.). Seattle, WA: University of Washington.
9. Rosenberg, H., Pollock, N., Schiemann, A. et al. (2015). Malignant hyperthermia: a review. *Orphanet J. Rare Dis.* 10: 93.
10. Rosenberg, H., Sambuughin, N., Riazi, S., and Dirksen, R. (1993). Malignant hyperthermia susceptibility. In: *GeneReviews®* (ed. M.P. Adam, H.H. Ardinger, R.A. Pagon, et al.). Seattle, WA: University of Washington.
11. Kraemer, K.H. and DiGiovanna, J.J. (1993). Xeroderma pigmentosum. In: *GeneReviews®* (ed. M.P. Adam, H.H. Ardinger, R.A. Pagon, et al.). Seattle, WA: University of Washington.
12. Clark, J.F. and Cecil, K.M. (2015). Diagnostic methods and recommendations for the cerebral creatine deficiency syndromes. *Pediatr. Res.* 77: 398–405.
13. Mercimek-Andrews, S. and Salomons, G.S. (1993). Creatine deficiency syndromes. In: *GeneReviews®* (ed. M.P. Adam, H.H. Ardinger, R.A. Pagon, et al.). Seattle, WA: University of Washington.
14. Murray, M.L., Pepin, M., Peterson, S., and Byers, P.H. (2014). Pregnancy-related deaths and complications in women with vascular Ehlers-Danlos syndrome. *Genet. Med.* 16: 874–880.

15. Byers, P.H. (1993). Vascular Ehlers-Danlos syndrome. In: *GeneReviews®* (ed. M.P. Adam, H.H. Ardinger, R.A. Pagon, et al.). Seattle, WA: University of Washington.

16. Toro, J.R., Nickerson, M.L., Wei, M.H. et al. (2003). Mutations in the fumarate hydratase gene cause hereditary leiomyomatosis and renal cell cancer in families in North America. *Am. J. Hum. Genet.* 73: 95–106.

17. Wei, M.H., Toure, O., Glenn, G.M. et al. (2006). Novel mutations in FH and expansion of the spectrum of phenotypes expressed in families with hereditary leiomyomatosis and renal cell cancer. *J. Med. Genet.* 43: 18–27.

18. Kamihara, J., Schultz, K.A., and Rana, H.Q. (1993). FH tumor predisposition syndrome. In: *GeneReviews®* (ed. M.P. Adam, H.H. Ardinger, R.A. Pagon, et al.). Seattle, WA: University of Washington.

19. Dunbar, C.E., High, K.A., Joung, J.K. et al. (2018). Gene therapy comes of age. *Science* 359.

20. High, K.A. and Roncarolo, M.G. (2019). Gene therapy. *N. Engl. J. Med.* 381: 455–464.

21. Nesterova, G. and Gahl, W.A. (2013). Cystinosis: the evolution of a treatable disease. *Pediatr. Nephrol.* 28: 51–59.

22. Nesterova, G. and Gahl, W.A. (1993). Cystinosis. In: *GeneReviews®* (ed. M.P. Adam, H.H. Ardinger, R.A. Pagon, et al.). Seattle, WA: University of Washington.

23. Zanger, U.M. and Schwab, M. (2013). Cytochrome P450 enzymes in drug metabolism: regulation of gene expression, enzyme activities, and impact of genetic variation. *Pharmacol. Ther.* 138: 103–141.

24. McCarthy, J.J. and Mendelsohn, B.A. (2017). *Precision Medicine: A Guide to Genomics in Clinical Practice*. New York: (McGraw Hill Professional).

25. Luzzatto, L. and Arese, P. (2018). Favism and glucose-6-phosphate dehydrogenase deficiency. *N. Engl. J. Med.* 378: 60–71.

26. Nussbaum, R.L., McInnes, R.R., and Willard, H.F. (2016). *Thompson & Thompson Genetics in Medicine*. Philadelphia, PA: Elsevier.

27. Yehia, L. and Eng, C. (1993). PTEN hamartoma tumor syndrome. In: *GeneReviews®* (ed. M.P. Adam, H.H. Ardinger, R.A. Pagon, et al.). Seattle, WA: University of Washington.

28. Gruters, A. and Krude, H. (2011). Detection and treatment of congenital hypothyroidism. *Nat. Rev. Endocrinol.* 8: 104–113.

29. Bodian, D.L., Klein, E., Iyer, R.K. et al. (2016). Utility of whole-genome sequencing for detection of newborn screening disorders in a population cohort of 1,696 neonates. *Genet. Med.* 18: 221–230.

30. Jaeger, B. and Bosch, A.M. (2016). Clinical presentation and outcome of riboflavin transporter deficiency: mini review after five years of experience. *J. Inherit. Metab. Dis.* 39: 559–564.

31. Barile, M., Giancaspero, T.A., Leone, P. et al. (2016). Riboflavin transport and metabolism in humans. *J. Inherit. Metab. Dis.* 39: 545–557.

32. Cali, E., Dominik, N., Manole, A., and Houlden, H. (1993). Riboflavin transporter deficiency. In: *GeneReviews®* (ed. M.P. Adam, H.H. Ardinger, R.A. Pagon, et al.). Seattle, WA: University of Washington.

33. Toriello, H.V. (2011). Thrombocytopenia-absent radius syndrome. *Semin. Thromb. Hemost.* 37: 707–712.

34. Albers, C.A., Paul, D.S., Schulze, H. et al. (2012). Compound inheritance of a low-frequency regulatory SNP and a rare null mutation in exon-junction complex subunit RBM8A causes TAR syndrome. *Nat. Genet.* 44 (435–439): S431–S432.

35. Stevenson, R.E., Allanson, J.G., Everman, D.B., and Solomon, B.D. (2016). *Human Malformations and Related Anomalies.* Oxford; New York: Oxford University Press).

36. Salvadori, M.I., Price, V.E., and Canadian Paediatric Society, Infectious Diseases and Immunization Committee (2014). Preventing and treating infections in children with asplenia or hyposplenia. *Paediatr. Child Health* 19: 271–278.

37. Bouteldja, N. and Timson, D.J. (2010). The biochemical basis of hereditary fructose intolerance. *J. Inherit. Metab. Dis.* 33: 105–112.

38. Demirbas, D., Brucker, W.J., and Berry, G.T. (2018). Inborn errors of metabolism with hepatopathy: metabolism defects of galactose, fructose, and tyrosine. *Pediatr. Clin. N. Am.* 65: 337–352.

39. Gaughan, S., Ayres, L., and Baker, P.R. II. (1993). Hereditary fructose intolerance. In: *GeneReviews®* (ed. M.P. Adam, H.H. Ardinger, R.A. Pagon, et al.). Seattle, WA: University of Washington.

40. Ah Mew, N., Simpson, K.L., Gropman, A.L. et al. (1993). Urea cycle disorders overview. In: *GeneReviews®* (ed. M.P. Adam, H.H. Ardinger, R.A. Pagon, et al.). Seattle, WA: University of Washington.

41. Haberle, J., Burlina, A., Chakrapani, A. et al. (2019). Suggested guidelines for the diagnosis and management of urea cycle disorders: first revision. *J. Inherit. Metab. Dis.* 42: 1192–1230.

42. Wolf, B. (2012). Biotinidase deficiency: "if you have to have an inherited metabolic disease, this is the one to have". *Genet. Med.* 14: 565–575.

43. Kury, S., Ramaekers, V., Bezieau, S., and Wolf, B. (2016). Clinical utility gene card for: Biotinidase deficiency-update 2015. *Eur. J. Hum. Genet.* 24.

44. Wolf, B. (1993). Biotinidase deficiency. In: *GeneReviews®* (ed. M.P. Adam, H.H. Ardinger, R.A. Pagon, et al.). Seattle, WA: University of Washington.

45. Lewis, R.A. (1993). Oculocutaneous albinism type 1 – retired chapter, for historical reference only. In: *GeneReviews®* (ed. M.P. Adam, H.H. Ardinger, R.A. Pagon, et al.). Seattle, WA: University of Washington.

46. Lewis, R.A. (1993). Ocular albinism, X-linked – retired chapter, for historical reference only. In: *GeneReviews®* (ed. M.P. Adam, H.H. Ardinger, R.A. Pagon, et al.). Seattle, WA: University of Washington.

47. Roizen, N.J. and Patterson, D. (2003). Down's syndrome. *Lancet* 361: 1281–1289.

48. Bull, M.J. and Committee on, G (2011). Health supervision for children with Down syndrome. *Pediatrics* 128: 393–406.

49. Parenti, G., Andria, G., and Ballabio, A. (2015). Lysosomal storage diseases: from pathophysiology to therapy. *Annu. Rev. Med.* 66: 471–486.

50. Cachon-Gonzalez, M.B., Zaccariotto, E., and Cox, T.M. (2018). Genetics and therapies for GM2 gangliosidosis. *Curr. Gene Ther.* 18: 68–89.

51. Flinn, A.M. and Gennery, A.R. (2018). Adenosine deaminase deficiency: a review. *Orphanet J. Rare Dis.* 13: 65.

52. Toro, C., Shirvan, L., and Tifft, C. (1993). HEXA disorders. In: *GeneReviews®* (ed. M.P. Adam, H.H. Ardinger, R.A. Pagon, et al.). Seattle, WA: University of Washington.

53. Jasperson, K.W., Patel, S.G., and Ahnen, D.J. (1993). APC-associated polyposis conditions. In: *GeneReviews®* (ed. M.P. Adam, H.H. Ardinger, R.A. Pagon, et al.). Seattle, WA: University of Washington.

Chapter 5

54. National comprehensive cancer network. https://www.nccn.org/professionals/physician_gls/pdf/genetics_colon.pdf (acessed 26 July 21).

55. Dietz, H. (1993). Marfan syndrome. In: *GeneReviews*® (ed. M.P. Adam, H.H. Ardinger, R.A. Pagon, et al.). Seattle, WA: University of Washington.

56. Milewicz, D.M., Braverman, A.C., De Backer, J. et al. (2021). Marfan syndrome. *Nat. Rev. Dis. Primers.* 7: 64.

57. King, M.C., Marks, J.H., Mandell, J.B., and New York Breast Cancer Study Group (2003). Breast and ovarian cancer risks due to inherited mutations in BRCA1 and BRCA2. *Science* 302: 643–646.

58. Litton, J.K., Rugo, H.S., Ettl, J. et al. (2018). Talazoparib in patients with advanced breast cancer and a germline BRCA mutation. *N. Engl. J. Med.* 379: 753–763.

59. Cheng, H.H., Sokolova, A.O., Schaeffer, E.M. et al. (2019). Germline and somatic mutations in prostate cancer for the clinician. *J. Natl. Compr. Cancer Netw.* 17: 515–521.

60. Mohyuddin, G.R., Aziz, M., Britt, A. et al. (2020). Similar response rates and survival with PARP inhibitors for patients with solid tumors harboring somatic versus Germline BRCA mutations: a meta-analysis and systematic review. *BMC Cancer* 20: 507.

61. Ellaway, C.J., Sholler, G., Leonard, H., and Christodoulou, J. (1999). Prolonged QT interval in Rett syndrome. *Arch. Dis. Child.* 80: 470–472.

62. Crosson, J., Srivastava, S., Bibat, G.M. et al. (2017). Evaluation of QTc in Rett syndrome: correlation with age, severity, and genotype. *Am. J. Med. Genet. A* 173: 1495–1501.

63. Kaur, S. and Christodoulou, J. (1993). MECP2 disorders. In: *GeneReviews*® (ed. M.P. Adam, H.H. Ardinger, R.A. Pagon, et al.). Seattle, WA: University of Washington.

64. Maude, S.L., Frey, N., Shaw, P.A. et al. (2014). Chimeric antigen receptor T cells for sustained remissions in leukemia. *N. Engl. J. Med.* 371: 1507–1517.

65. Maude, S.L., Laetsch, T.W., Buechner, J. et al. (2018). Tisagenlecleucel in children and young adults with B-cell lymphoblastic leukemia. *N. Engl. J. Med.* 378: 439–448.

66. Mills, P.B., Struys, E., Jakobs, C. et al. (2006). Mutations in antiquitin in individuals with pyridoxine-dependent seizures. *Nat. Med.* 12: 307–309.

67. Olson, H.E., Poduri, A., and Pearl, P.L. (2014). Genetic forms of epilepsies and other paroxysmal disorders. *Semin. Neurol.* 34: 266–279.

68. Coughlin, C.R. 2nd, Tseng, L.A., Abdenur, J.E. et al. (2021). Consensus guidelines for the diagnosis and management of pyridoxine-dependent epilepsy due to alpha-aminoadipic semialdehyde dehydrogenase deficiency. *J. Inherit. Metab. Dis.* 44: 178–192.

Inheritance, Risk, and Related Calculations

6

6.1. A child has severe, autosomal recessive neonatal disorder. What's the chance his healthy five-year-old sister is a carrier?

A. 5%

B. 25%

C. 50%

D. 67%

6.2. What inheritance pattern is most likely in the pedigree shown below?

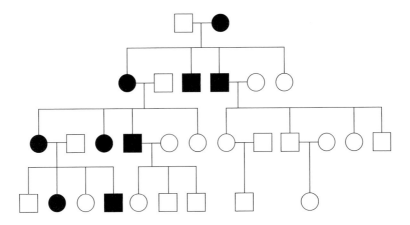

A. Autosomal recessive

B. X-linked dominant

C. X-linked recessive

D. Mitochondrial

6.3. Assuming Hardy-Weinberg Equilibrium (HWE), if 100 people in a population of 1 million have an autosomal recessive disorder, how many heterozygous carriers are there expected to be in that population?

A. 10

B. 1000

C. 20 000

D. 200 000

6.4. An adult has non-insulin-dependent diabetes mellitus. She does not have a strong family history of this condition but has other risks, such as her weight. In general, according to current knowledge, what is the best description of this condition from an etiologic/genetic perspective?

A. Autosomal dominant

B. Epigenetic

C. Multifactorial

D. X-linked

Medical Genetics and Genomics: Questions for Board Review, First Edition. Benjamin D. Solomon.
© 2023 John Wiley & Sons Ltd. Published 2023 by John Wiley & Sons Ltd.

6.5. A woman is a carrier for a pathogenic variant for an X-linked recessive disorder. What is the chance that her next child will have the disorder?

A. 5%   C. 33%

B. 25%   D. 50%

6.6. A set of DNA variants along one chromosome are found to be inherited together in different people (all of the tested people have the same variants). How might this set of genetic changes be described?

A. Codon   C. Locus

B. Haplotype   D. Telomere

6.7. Approximately what percent of Down syndrome is sporadic, due to nonfamilial trisomy 21?

A. 5%   C. 95%

B. 50%   D. 100%

6.8. Which of the conditions below has an X-linked inheritance pattern?

A. Achondroplasia   C. Huntington disease

B. Hemophilia A   D. Sickle cell anemia

6.9. Currently, about what percent of breast cancer in women is thought to be due to relatively high-penetrance germline pathogenic variants?

A. <1%   C. 50–75%

B. 5–10%   D. >90%

6.10. What is the inheritance of heritable retinoblastoma at the family level (i.e. what inheritance pattern would a pedigree of the family be expected to show)?

A. Autosomal dominant   C. Mitochondrial

B. Autosomal recessive   D. X-linked dominant

6.11. A family is affected by a rare autosomal dominant condition. What is the chance that a grandchild of an affected person will have the condition?

A. 25%   C. 75%

B. 50%   D. 100%

6.12. Which "repeat disorder" involves autosomal recessive inheritance?

A. Fragile X syndrome   C. Huntington disease

B. Friedreich ataxia   D. Myotonic dystrophy

6.13. Pathogenic variants in what gene appear to result in the highest risk of male breast cancer?

A. *BRCA1*   C. *CHEK2*

B. *BRCA2*   D. *PALB2*

6.14. An apparently healthy adult woman is referred to genetics because her father and sister have what appears to be a type of familial hypertrophic cardiomyopathy. Who would be the most informative family member to test first?

A. The woman's child   C. The woman herself

B. The woman's father   D. The woman's mother

6.15. Approximately what percentage of infants in the United States are affected by birth defects?

A. 0.1–0.5%   C. 10–15%
B. 2–3%   D. 18–20%

6.16. Which of the following images best depicts monozygotic twins, both of whom are affected by the same condition?

(a)    (b)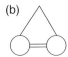

(c)    (d)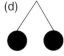

6.17. A child has a genetic condition; genetic testing identifies an extremely rare pathogenic variant that appears to explain the presence of the genetic condition in the child. The parents are tested; neither appears to harbor the variant. Later, they have another child with the same condition and variant. Which of the following are possible explanations (though some may be more likely than others)?

A. Germline mosaicism   C. Testing error
B. Nonpaternity   D. All of the above

6.18. A woman and a man have a child. The man has another child with the woman's sister. Approximately what proportion of their DNA would the two children have in common?

A. 12.5%   C. 50%
B. 37.5%   D. 67%

6.19. A person is the only one in their family affected by a genetic condition. Genetic testing shows that the condition is due to a de novo pathogenic variant. Based on this information, which condition is LEAST likely to be affecting this person?

A. Achondroplasia   C. Marfan syndrome
B. Cystic fibrosis   D. Neurofibromatosis type 1

6.20. A person would be expected to have the lowest proportion of DNA in common with which relative?

A. Child   C. Grandparent
B. First cousin   D. Half-sibling

6.21. An apparently healthy adult woman was referred to genetics because her father and sister have familial hypertrophic cardiomyopathy. Genetic testing reveals a variant of uncertain significance (VUS) in a relevant gene in the father, which is not resolved by further familial testing. Based on this, what is recommended for the woman?

A. Discharge from care

B. Genetic testing of her children

C. Immediate ICD placement

D. Regular clinical cardiac evaluation

6.22. Which of the following conditions is most likely to be depicted in the pedigree shown?

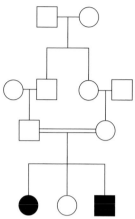

A. Duchenne muscular dystrophy

B. Fabry disease

C. Loeys-Dietz syndrome

D. Propionic acidemia

6.23. A male patient has an X-linked condition. Which other relative could also have the same condition?

A. His father

B. His maternal uncle

C. His paternal uncle

D. His son

6.24. Which of the following are generally considered to be as genetically similar as siblings?

A. Dizygotic twins

B. First cousins

C. Half-siblings

D. Monozygotic twins

6.25. Multiple siblings in a family have a rare genetic condition. Which of the following would most suggest autosomal recessive inheritance?

A. Anticipation

B. Congenital onset

C. Consanguinity

D. Only males are affected

6.26. What is the term for the inheritance of two copies of a chromosome or part of a chromosome from one parent (and no copies from the other parent)?

A. Mosaicism

B. Recombination

C. Uniparental disomy

D. X-linked inheritance

6.27. As a genetic change is "passed down" within a family, the related condition is observed to appear at an earlier age and with more severe clinical findings. Which of the following describes this observation?

A. Anticipation

B. Incomplete penetrance

C. Nonsense-mediated decay

D. Variable expressivity

6.28. A neonate has an older brother with molecularly confirmed familial Hemophagocytic lymphohistiocytosis (fHLH). Based on the causes of fHLH, what is the most likely chance that the neonate will also be "genetically affected" (will have also inherited the causative variant(s))?
A. 25%
B. 33%
C. 50%
D. 67%

6.29. A large family has multiple members who have had cancer. Many affected family members have a pathogenic variant in *BRCA1*. However, one individual, who had early-onset breast cancer, does not have this variant. What is the best term for this individual/phenomenon?
A. Carrier
B. Hemizygous
C. Nonpenetrant
D. Phenocopy

6.30. A person has type AB blood. This is because two phenotypes are expressed from the same gene (each allele is expressed). What is the best description for the inheritance that explains this phenotype?
A. Autosomal dominant
B. Codominant
C. Incompletely dominant
D. Semidominant

6.31. A man and a woman are seen together for prenatal counseling. The couple, both of whom are healthy, are from a community where a childhood-onset autosomal recessive genetic condition affects about 1 in 100 people. The man's brother has the condition. What is the approximate chance that the couple's child will be affected?
A. 0.1%
B. 1%
C. 3%
D. 6%

6.32. A patient diagnosed with cancer in early adulthood undergoes germline genetic testing; the result is a variant of uncertain significance (VUS). Testing which of the following individuals would be LEAST likely to be informative related to variant pathogenicity?
A. Affected older sibling
B. Affected parent
C. Unaffected child
D. Unaffected parent

6.33. Which term refers to a combined risk that is calculated by aggregating the contributions of multiple different genetic changes to a condition or disease?
A. Carrier risk
B. LOD score
C. Polygenic risk score
D. Relative risk

6.34. A woman's mother is a carrier for a severe X-linked recessive condition; the woman has an affected brother. The woman also has two unaffected sons. What is the chance that she is a carrier?
A. 1/10
B. 1/5
C. 1/4
D. 1/2

6.35. Prenatal ultrasound shows findings consistent with Thanataphoric dysplasia; molecular testing via amniocentesis confirms the diagnosis. No parental testing has been done yet. What is the most likely recurrence risk based on this information?
A. <1%
B. 25%
C. 33%
D. 50%

6.36. A patient has an autosomal recessive genetic condition. You notice that there are many reported pathogenic variants in the relevant gene; none are common in any population. Based on this, the patient would probably be (regarding the causative variants in this gene):

A. Compound heterozygous   **C.** Isodisomic

B. Homozygous   **D.** Mosaic

6.37. A man and a woman have two children, both of whom are affected by an autosomal recessive condition. The woman is pregnant; what is the chance that their next child will be a boy with this condition?

A. 0.5%   **C.** 25%

B. 12.5%   **D.** 33%

6.38. An apparently healthy woman gives birth to a term male infant. Her brother had a severe inborn error of metabolism, and testing shows that her newborn son is also affected. Assuming no consanguinity or other such circumstance, what condition is most likely in this family?

A. Biotinidase deficiency   **C.** Phenylketonuria

B. Ornithine transcarbamylase deficiency   **D.** Wilson disease

6.39. Which inheritance pattern is most likely in the pedigree shown below?

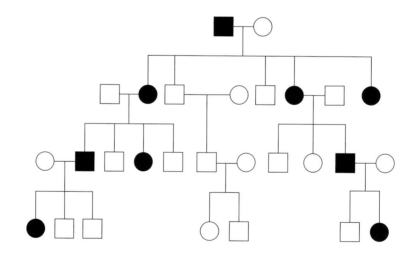

A. Autosomal dominant   **C.** X-linked dominant

B. Autosomal recessive   **D.** X-linked recessive

6.40. A woman is affected by an autosomal dominant condition (that is completely penetrant). She has three children. What is the chance that all three of her children are affected by the condition?

A. 12.5%   **C.** 50%

B. 25%   **D.** 75%

Answers

6.1.	D	6.11.	A	6.21.	D	6.31.	C
6.2.	D	6.12.	B	6.22.	D	6.32.	C
6.3.	C	6.13.	B	6.23.	B	6.33.	C
6.4.	C	6.14.	B	6.24.	A	6.34.	B
6.5.	B	6.15.	B	6.25.	C	6.35.	A
6.6.	B	6.16.	C	6.26.	C	6.36.	A
6.7.	C	6.17.	D	6.27.	A	6.37.	B
6.8.	B	6.18.	B	6.28.	A	6.38.	B
6.9.	B	6.19.	B	6.29.	D	6.39.	C
6.10.	A	6.20.	B	6.30.	B	6.40.	A

Chapter 6

Commentary

6.1. *67%*

For this question, it may help to look at a pedigree and Punnett square (see below). For the sake of simplicity here (as with the other questions in this book), we will assume there are no "real life" complicating circumstances such as incomplete penetrance, nonbiological parentage (e.g. nonpaternity), etc. For the autosomal recessive disease described, the affected child would be homozygous for the disease-causing variant (a); her genotype would be written as: aa. Each parent would be a carrier; their genotypes would each be: Aa. The healthy older sister could not be aa. We know this because she is a healthy five year-old and this is a severe neonatal condition. Thus, the older sister could either be AA or Aa. From the Punnet square, there are two possibilities for her to be Aa and one possibility be AA, so there is a ⅔ (67%) chance the healthy older sister is a carrier (Aa). The key thing to remember is that the healthy sister cannot have the aa genotype.

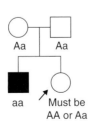
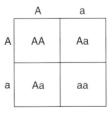

Reference(s): Nussbaum et al. [1].

6.2. Mitochondrial

The most important clue that this pedigree represents mitochondrial inheritance is that only mothers pass on the condition to their children. That is, the condition is only maternally inherited. There are several points worth noting. First, some mitochondrial conditions can have "nuclear" (e.g. autosomal recessive) inheritance – these are conditions that involve mitochondrial function but where the gene is part of the nuclear DNA rather than the mitochondrial DNA. Second, in a condition with mitochondrial inheritance, children of an affected mother may or may not be clinically affected, and there can be variable expressivity. This has to do with factors such as the proportion of variant-positive mitochondrial DNA passed down to the child and the proportion of variant-positive mitochondrial DNA present in the child's different tissues. The condition shown in the pedigree is unlikely to be autosomal recessive because affected individuals have affected children, but this could theoretically be possible if variants in the associated gene were very common in the population shown on the pedigree. The condition is not X-linked dominant because the daughters of affected males are unaffected. The condition is not X-linked recessive because females are affected. However, there are "real life" exceptions to the rules about these inheritance patterns, and many pedigrees will not yield obvious clues as to the inheritance pattern, including because there may not be enough information regarding many relatives.

Reference(s): Chinnery [2]; Nussbaum et al. [1].

6.3. 20 000

From the question, we know that 100 people out of the population of 1 000 000 have the autosomal recessive disease mentioned. Using the standard abbreviations, this means that the frequency of affected individuals, those with two copies of the disease-causing allele (q^2) is 100/1 000 000 or 0.0001. The frequency of the q allele is the square root of 0.0001, or 0.01. The frequency of the p allele, the wild-type or normal allele, is $1-q$ or $1-0.01$, which is 0.99. The frequency of heterozygotes, who have one normal and one disease-related allele, is 2pq or (2)(0.99)(0.01), which equals 0.0198. Last, to get the number of heterozygotes, we multiply the frequency of heterozygotes by the population: (0.0198) (1 000 000), which equals 19 800.

Reference(s): Nussbaum et al. [1].

6.4. Multifactorial

Medical conditions and other phenotypes can have a variety of causes. The cause of some genetic conditions is known and may follow a recognized inheritance pattern. Many medical conditions do not have clear genetic causes and may result from a complex interplay of genetic and nongenetic factors; one term for this is multifactorial.

Reference(s): Nussbaum et al. [1]; van Tilburg et al. [3]; Morris [4].

6.5. 25%

The woman is a carrier for a pathogenic variant related to an X-linked recessive disorder; her genotype could be abbreviated as $X^A X^a$, where X^A indicates the wild-type allele and X^a indicates the allele with the pathogenic variant. Let us assume her partner's genotype is X^{A}Y, although there may be exceptions. There are then generally four possibilities for her children: X^{A}X^A (a female who is not a carrier); X^{A}X^a (a carrier female); X^{A}Y (an unaffected male); X^{a}Y (an affected male). There is therefore a 1 in 4 or 25% chance that her next child will have the disorder. If, for example, the question had asked "what is the chance that her next son will have the disorder?", the answer would be 50%.

Reference(s): Nussbaum et al. [1].

6.6. Haplotype

A haplotype is a term that describes a group of DNA variants that are typically inherited together because they are located close to each other on a chromosome. Knowledge of relevant haplotypes can be important in both research and clinical settings.

Reference(s): International HapMap Consortium [5].

6.7. 95%

Approximately 95% of Down syndrome occurs sporadically, and is termed nonfamilial trisomy 21. In about 3–4%, the extra chromosomal material is due to an unbalanced translocation between chromosome 21 and another acrocentric chromosome. Of these unbalanced translocations, about 75% are de novo, and about 25% are familial translocations. In about 1–2% of people with the Down syndrome phenotype, there is mosaicism for euploid cell line and one cell line with trisomy 21.

Reference(s): Roizen and Patterson [6]; Bull et al. [7].

6.8. Hemophilia A

Hemophilia A is an X-linked bleeding disorder due to pathogenic variants in *F8*, resulting in deficient factor VIII clotting activity. This deficiency leads to clinical manifestations such as prolonged bleeding after injuries, minor trauma, surgery, or dental extractions. Hemophilia B, which involves factor IX deficiency, is also X-linked.

Reference(s): Konkle et al. [8].

6.9. 5–10%

About 5–10% of breast cancer in women is currently believed to be due to relatively high-penetrance germline pathogenic variants. However, this is an extremely active area of investigation. Newly contributory genes and variants, as well as more complicated models of causation, are continually being identified and analyzed, including through studies of larger and more diverse groups of individuals.

Reference(s): Newman et al. [9]; Pharoah et al. [10]; Foulkes [11]; Buys et al. [12]; Couch et al. [13].

6.10. Autosomal dominant

Heritable retinoblastoma is caused by pathogenic variants in the gene *RB1*. These can be inherited in an autosomal dominant manner, but can also occur de novo. In heritable retinoblastoma, in addition to the heterozygous *RB1* pathogenic variant, retinoblastoma occurs when another pathogenic variant affects the other allele - this is sometimes referred to as the "two-hit" model of disease. In addition to retinoblastoma, patients are also at higher risk of other, non-ophthalmologic tumors.

Reference(s): Knudson [14]; Lohmann and Gallie [15].

6.11. 25%

The question refers to a rare condition, so we will assume an affected person is heterozygous for the causative allele. We can represent the genotype of an affected person as: Dd. D represents the dominant allele (in this case, the version of the gene that has the disease-causing genetic change) and d represents the recessive allele (in this case, the version of the gene that does not have the disease-causing genetic change). The child of each affected person has a 50% chance of inheriting the dominant allele (D). The question is about a grandchild being affected. From the question, we don't know if that grandchild's parent has the condition or not. In other words, since there are two generations, the chance of a grandchild inheriting the dominant allele and having the condition = $(\frac{1}{2})(\frac{1}{2}) = \frac{1}{4}$ or 25%.

Reference(s): Nussbaum et al. [1].

6.12. Friedreich ataxia

Friedreich ataxia (FRDA) is an autosomal recessive, progressive neurological disorder with a mean age of onset of 10–15 years. Manifestations commonly include gait and limb ataxia with associated muscle weakness, absent lower limb reflexes, dysarthria, and loss of vibratory sense and proprioception. Other features can include cardiomyopathy and diabetes mellitus. FRDA is most commonly caused by expansion of a GAA trinucleotide repeat in intron 1 of the *FXN* gene.

Reference(s): Bidichandani and Delatycki [16]; Paulson [17].

6.13. *BRCA2*

Pathogenic variants in *BRCA2* confer an elevated risk for different types of cancer, including breast, melanoma, ovarian, prostate, and pancreatic cancer. The cumulative risk for men with *BRCA2* pathogenic variants is about 7% by 70 years of age (one study showed a cumulative risk of about 9% by 80 years of age). Male breast cancer accounts for less than 1% of all breast cancer.

Reference(s): Tai et al. [18]; Evans et al. [19]; Petrucelli et al. [20]; Giordano [21].

6.14. The woman's father

In this question, we know that the father and sister have familial hypertrophic cardiomyopathy, but the genetic cause has not yet been identified. The woman may have been referred because she has concerns about her health or that of other family members who may be affected (such as her children). In this situation, although the woman is described as healthy, we do not know whether she harbors a pathogenic variant that may be causing the condition in her father and sister. Genetic testing of her father (or sister) might identify the genetic cause in the family, which could potentially allow genetic testing in other family members to be considered at that point. If one were to start by testing the woman herself (prior to testing family members who are clearly affected), interpreting the results might be more difficult.

Reference(s): Nussbaum et al. [1]; Cirino and Ho [22].

6.15. 2–3%

About 2–3% of infants born in the United States are affected by birth defects (congenital anomalies), or structural changes that can affect different parts of the body. There are many different types of birth defects, and the severity can vary considerably. The causes of some birth defects are understood, but for others, the causes remain unclear. Birth defects contribute very significantly to infant morbidity and mortality.

Reference(s): Centers for Disease Control and Prevention (CDC) [23]; Feldkamp et al. [24].

6.16.

Choice C (the image shown above) depicts monozygotic (identical) female twins, both affected by the same condition. The fact that they are monozygotic is shown by the bar connecting the two lines extending to each of the two individuals. They are both "colored in," which implies that they are both affected by the condition in question.

Reference(s): Gonzaga-Jauregui and Lupski [25]; Bennett et al. [26].

6.17. All of the above

A child has an apparently de novo variant; later, a sibling is born with the same variant. There are multiple possible explanations. First, nonpaternity is possible, though would have to involve the same partner both times (as the variant is extremely rare), and lab testing could confirm biological parentage. Second, some type of testing error is possible, though the chance of this happening can again be reduced with steps such as confirmation of sample identity and biological parentage as well as other safeguards. Third, germline (gonadal) mosaicism may occur, in which one of the parents harbors the causative variant in the germline (sperm or egg), but not in the tissue (e.g. a blood sample) that was tested for the presence of the variant in question.

Reference(s): Gonzaga-Jauregui and Lupski [25]; Nussbaum et al. [1].

6.18. 37.5%

On average, full siblings have about 50% of their DNA in common. Half-siblings share about 25% of their DNA in common. In this question, however, the children have the same father and their mothers are sisters; these children have been termed "three-quarter siblings." These children would be expected, on average, to share about 37.5% of their DNA.

Reference(s): Galván-Femenía et al. [27].

6.19. Cystic fibrosis

People affected by genetic conditions may be the first person in a family who is known to be affected by a particular genetic condition. There are multiple different reasons for this. For example, some people with certain conditions, such as achondroplasia, Marfan syndrome, and neurofibromatosis type one, may have the condition due to dominantly inherited pathogenic variants in the corresponding genes. These conditions can also arise due to de novo pathogenic variants. Cystic fibrosis, on the other hand, is an autosomal recessive condition, and the condition is much less likely to involve de novo variants.

Reference(s): White et al. [28]; Saranjam et al. [29]; Ong et al. [30].

6.20. First cousin

The proportion of DNA a person shares with their relatives depends on how closely the individuals are related. A person shares approximately 50% of their DNA with a child, approximately 25% with a grandparent or half-sibling, and approximately 12.5% with a first cousin.

Reference(s): Nussbaum et al. [1].

6.21. Regular clinical cardiac evaluation

In the description of the family, a variant of uncertain significance (VUS) has been identified, but its pathogenicity has not been resolved by further familial testing. Based on this information, the woman would be advised to continue to undergo regular clinical cardiac evaluation; this evaluation plan would likely be tailored to the specific genetic condition and family history. Clinical findings (e.g. if cardiac testing were to identify signs of cardiomyopathy) would be treated accordingly. If a pathogenic variant explaining the condition were found in the affected members of the family, and the woman were found not to have the variant, she could be dismissed from care.

Reference(s): Cirino and Ho [22]; Nussbaum et al. [1].

6.22. Propionic acidemia

The pedigree shows what is likely to be an autosomal recessive condition, such as Propionic acidemia (the only autosomal recessive condition of the choices given). Hints that this is autosomal recessive include that nobody is affected in the family prior to the two children in the youngest generation, that both a male and a female are affected, and the relatedness of the parents of the affected children (the parents are first cousins).

Reference(s): Nussbaum et al. [1].

6.23. His maternal uncle

The figure may help explain this question. The proband (the affected male) is indicated with an arrow. In this theoretical scenario, his mother is a carrier for the X-linked genetic change. His maternal uncle could be affected, as he may also have inherited the same genetic change as the proband (from the proband's maternal grandmother, who is not pictured). The proband's father, son, and paternal uncle could not be affected, as they could not have the same X-linked genetic change – they cannot inherit the X-chromosome with the affected allele.

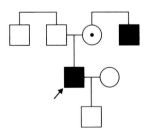

Reference(s): Nussbaum et al. [1].

6.24. Dizygotic twins

Dizygotic twins arise from two ova that have been independently fertilized by two different sperm. Thus, dizygotic twins are generally about as genetically similar as siblings.

Reference(s): Stevenson et al. [31].

6.25. Consanguinity

Consanguinity describes a union in which the parents are closely related to each other. Traditionally, in clinical genetics, this has been used to indicate unions of people who are related as second cousins or closer. Due to a larger proportion of shared genetic material among the parents, the offspring of their union are typically more likely to be affected by autosomal recessive conditions than if the parents were less related.

Reference(s): Alkuraya [32]; Solomon and Muenke [33]; Bhinder et al. [34].

6.26. Uniparental disomy

Uniparental disomy refers to the situation where two copies of a chromosome or part of a chromosome are inherited from one parent and no copies are inherited from the other parent. Uniparental disomy can cause disease in several possible ways, including by resulting in homozygosity for a pathogenic variant or by affecting imprinting.

Reference(s): Lapunzina and Monk [35]; Soellner et al. [36].

6.27. Anticipation

Anticipation refers to the phenomenon where a genetic condition can be more severe and appear at a younger age as the causative genetic change is passed down in a family. This can be observed in "repeat disorders," in which the number of repetitive sequences can expand as the gene is passed down. Examples of conditions in which anticipation may be observed include Myotonic dystrophy and Huntington disease.

Reference(s): Nussbaum et al. [1].

6.28. 25%

Familial Hemophagocytic lymphohistiocytosis (fHLH) is an autosomal recessive immunologic disorder that can be caused by pathogenic variants in multiple known genes. The history of an older affected sibling means that this infant would be expected to have a 25% chance of also being affected. fHLH typically presents with fever, hepatosplenomegaly, and cytopenia. Accurate diagnosis is important for management.

Reference(s): Zhang et al. [37].

6.29. Phenocopy

The term phenocopy can be used to describe a person who does not have a particular genetic change, but who has clinical findings that would make it seem like they "should have" that genetic change. In the example in the question, the person with early-onset breast cancer might be anticipated to have the *BRCA1* pathogenic variant found in the other family members but does not; that is, the person would have breast cancer due to causes other than the *BRCA1* variant.

Reference(s): NCI Dictionary of Genetic Terms [38].

6.30. Codominant

The term codominant refers to the phenomenon where two phenotypes are expressed from the same gene. Another way to describe this is that both alleles (both versions of the gene) are expressed in the heterozygote. In a person with type AB blood, they are heterozygous for two different alleles of the ABO gene. In this person, one allele causes the "A" molecule to be expressed on the surface of the red blood cells, while the other allele causes the "B" molecule to be expressed on the surface of the red blood cell. Thus, both alleles are expressed in this person.

Reference(s): Yamamoto et al. [39].

6.31. 3%

Chapter 6

Several calculations have to be made to arrive at the answer. There are some shortcuts/estimates that can be made to arrive at an estimate, but for the sake of education, we will not use these shortcuts in the explanation. First, we know that the man has a brother who has the condition. The man is healthy, so he does not have the condition. There is therefore a ⅔ chance he is a carrier, and a ⅓ chance he is not a carrier (if we didn't know whether he was affected, there would be a ½ (50%) chance he would be a carrier, but we know his clinical status, so we can eliminate the possibility that he is affected when doing the calculation). The condition affects 1/100 people in the population, so the frequency of the recessive allele (q) is 1/10, while the frequency of the wild-type allele (p) is 9/10. We estimate the prevalence of carriers as 2pq or $(2)(9/10)(1/10) = 18/100$. However, just to be precise, since we know that the woman does not have the condition, we can say that the chance of her being a carrier is 18/99. This is the same kind of adjustment we made previously, though it does not affect the final result very much, and often won't be necessary to arrive at a final estimate in this type of calculation. Now, we know that the chance of the man being a carrier is ⅔ and the chance of the woman being a carrier is 18/99. The chance of them both passing the affected alleles on to their child is ¼. Finally, we multiply these three fractions together to get the final answer: $(⅔)(18/99)(¼) = 0.0303$ or approximately 3%.

Reference(s): Nussbaum et al. [1].

6.32. Unaffected child

A variant of uncertain significance (VUS) refers to a genetic variant where the evidence of pathogenicity is unclear or incomplete. That is, it is unknown whether the VUS contributes to a particular disease, and it is recommended that a VUS not be used for clinical decision-making. To better understand whether the VUS contributes to disease in a person, various strategies can be used. One such strategy involves familial testing: testing of other relatives to see whether they have the VUS in question. When this is done in the context of gathering more information to evaluate a variant, it is important to consider which individuals may be informative in terms of contributing useful data. In the question given, knowing that the older sibling and mother are affected – and that the father is unaffected – can be helpful to determine whether the VUS in question segregates with affected status in the family (whether the VUS "tracks" with the presence of disease in the family). Testing the unaffected child of the patient may not be informative – for example, the child may simply be too young to be affected by the cancer seen in the patient.

Reference(s): Richards et al. [40]; Tsai et al. [41].

6.33. Polygenic risk score

A polygenic risk score refers to a mathematical score that is constructed to try to determine the risk of a condition or disorder. This score combines the contributions of multiple individual variants to estimate the chance of having the condition in question. Polygenic risk scores have been investigated for many conditions and in some cases are being studied or implemented in clinical settings.

Reference(s): Torkamani et al. [42]; Sugrue and Desikan [43].

6.34. 1/5

This question can be solved using a Bayesian analysis. The calculation for this question is shown in the table below:

Hypothesis	Carrier	Noncarrier
Prior probability	½	½
Conditional probability (of having two unaffected sons)	¼	~1
Joint probability	$(½)(¼) = ⅛$	$(½)(1) = ½$
Posterior probability	$(⅛)/(⅛ + ½) = ⅕$	$(½)/(⅛ + ½) = ⅘$

Based on the fact that her mother is a carrier, we know that the woman in the question started with a ½ (50%) chance of being a carrier and the same chance of not being a carrier; this is the prior probability in the table above. Next, if she were a carrier, her chance of having two unaffected sons would be (½)(½) or ¼ (25%); if she were not a carrier, her chance of having two unaffected sons would be approximately 1 (100%). This is the conditional probability. We calculate the joint probability for each possibility as the product of the prior and conditional probabilities. Finally, the posterior probability is the chance that each hypothesis is true after taking into account both the prior (original) and subsequent information. To calculate the posterior probability for each probability, one divides the joint probability for each hypothesis by the sum of the joint probabilities for each of the hypotheses (in this example, there are two hypotheses). For this question, we end up with a posterior probability of ⅕ (20%) for the hypothesis of her being a carrier given all the information we have.

Reference(s): Ogino and Wilson [44].

6.35. <1%

Thanataphoric dysplasia (TD) is a severe type of skeletal dysplasia, and is caused by heterozygous pathogenic variants in *FGFR3*. These variants usually occur de novo (though there is a theoretical possibility of issues such as germline mosaicism or other unusual situations that would affect the recurrence risk in a given situation). As the variants usually occur de novo, the risk to a subsequent conception would be about the same as in the general population, or far less than 1%.

Reference(s): Schild et al. [45]; French and Savarirayan [46].

6.36. Compound heterozygous

A patient with an autosomal recessive genetic condition will have two pathogenic variants, one on each allele. That is, this person will have biallelic pathogenic variants. In a situation where it is likely that these two variants are different, the individual would have compound heterozygous pathogenic variants in the involved gene. (As with just about everything in genetics, there are of course rare exceptions.)

Reference(s): Nussbaum et al. [1].

6.37. 12.5%

In the question, both parents are presumed to be heterozygous "carriers" for a pathogenic variant in the relevant gene. Except for certain unusual circumstances, the chance that any one of their children will be affected is 25%. This does not depend on the number of previously affected or unaffected children. Again, assuming that there are no unusual circumstances, the chance for a child to be a boy is approximately 50%. Thus, the chance for the next child to be an affected boy= 25% × 50% = (0.25)(0.5) = 0.125 or 12.5%.

Reference(s): Nussbaum et al. [1].

6.38. Ornithine transcarbamylase deficiency

Ornithine transcarbamylase (OTC) deficiency, caused by pathogenic variants in *OTC*, is an X-linked urea cycle disorder. In the question, the history of the affected brother, the apparently healthy mother (the sister of the affected brother), and the newborn son with the same condition as his uncle, suggest an X-linked condition. Of note, it is estimated that approximately 20–30% of females harboring pathogenic variants in OTC will display some clinical manifestations. Early diagnosis is important for acute and chronic treatment.

Reference(s): Gyato et al. [47]; Lichter-Konecki et al. [48]; Kalia et al. [49].

6.39. X-linked dominant

The pedigree depicts X-linked dominant inheritance. Hints that X-linked dominant inheritance is involved include the fact that affected fathers have all affected daughters and no affected sons, and that affected daughters can have affected or unaffected sons and daughters. It can be difficult to differentiate autosomal dominant from X-linked dominant inheritance, especially in a small pedigree.

Reference(s): Nussbaum et al. [1].

6.40. 12.5%

The woman has an autosomal dominant condition; each of her children has a 50% (0.5) chance of inheriting the causative allele. Since she has three children, the chance of all of them being affected can be calculated as (0.5)(0.5)(0.5) = 0.125 or 12.5%.

Reference(s): Nussbaum et al. [1].

References

1. Nussbaum, R.L., McInnes, R.R., and Willard, H.F. (2016). *Thompson & Thompson Genetics in Medicine*. Philadelphia, PA: Elsevier.
2. Chinnery, P.F. (1993). Primary mitochondrial disorders overview. In: *GeneReviews®* (ed. M.P. Adam, H.H. Ardinger, R.A. Pagon, et al.). Seattle, WA: University of Washington.

3. van Tilburg, J., van Haeften, T.W., Pearson, P., and Wijmenga, C. (2001). Defining the genetic contribution of type 2 diabetes mellitus. *J. Med. Genet.* 38: 569–578.

4. Morris, A.P. (2018). Progress in defining the genetic contribution to type 2 diabetes susceptibility. *Curr. Opin. Genet. Dev.* 50: 41–51.

5. The International HapMap Consortium (2005). A haplotype map of the human genome. *Nature* 437: 1299–1320.

6. Roizen, N.J. and Patterson, D. (2003). Down's syndrome. *Lancet* 361: 1281–1289.

7. Bull, M.J. and Committee on, G (2011). Health supervision for children with Down syndrome. *Pediatrics* 128: 393–406.

8. Konkle, B.A., Huston, H., and Nakaya Fletcher, S. (1993). Hemophilia A. In: *GeneReviews*® (ed. M.P. Adam, H.H. Ardinger, R.A. Pagon, et al.). Seattle (WA): University of Washington.

9. Newman, B., Austin, M.A., Lee, M., and King, M.C. (1988). Inheritance of human breast cancer: evidence for autosomal dominant transmission in high-risk families. *Proc. Natl Acad. Sci. USA* 85: 3044–3048.

10. Pharoah, P.D., Antoniou, A., Bobrow, M. et al. (2002). Polygenic susceptibility to breast cancer and implications for prevention. *Nat. Genet.* 31: 33–36.

11. Foulkes, W.D. (2008). Inherited susceptibility to common cancers. *N. Engl. J. Med.* 359: 2143–2153.

12. Buys, S.S., Sandbach, J.F., Gammon, A. et al. (2017). A study of over 35,000 women with breast cancer tested with a 25-gene panel of hereditary cancer genes. *Cancer* 123: 1721–1730.

13. Couch, F.J., Shimelis, H., Hu, C. et al. (2017). Associations between cancer predisposition testing panel genes and breast cancer. *JAMA Oncol.* 3: 1190–1196.

14. Knudson, A.G. Jr. (1971). Mutation and cancer: statistical study of retinoblastoma. *Proc. Natl Acad. Sci. USA* 68: 820–823.

15. Lohmann, D.R. and Gallie, B.L. (1993). Retinoblastoma. In: *GeneReviews*® (ed. M.P. Adam, H.H. Ardinger, R.A. Pagon, et al.). Seattle, WA: University of Washington.

16. Bidichandani, S.I. and Delatycki, M.B. (1993). Friedreich ataxia. In: *GeneReviews*® (ed. M.P. Adam, H.H. Ardinger, R.A. Pagon, et al.). Seattle, WA: University of Washington.

17. Paulson, H. (2018). Repeat expansion diseases. *Handb. Clin. Neurol.* 147: 105–123.

18. Tai, Y.C., Domchek, S., Parmigiani, G., and Chen, S. (2007). Breast cancer risk among male BRCA1 and BRCA2 mutation carriers. *J. Natl. Cancer Inst.* 99: 1811–1814.

19. Evans, D.G., Susnerwala, I., Dawson, J. et al. (2010). Risk of breast cancer in male BRCA2 carriers. *J. Med. Genet.* 47: 710–711.

20. Petrucelli, N., Daly, M.B., and Pal, T. (1993). BRCA1- and BRCA2-associated hereditary breast and ovarian cancer. In: *GeneReviews*® (ed. M.P. Adam, H.H. Ardinger, R.A. Pagon, et al.). Seattle, WA: University of Washington.

21. Giordano, S.H. (2018). Breast cancer in men. *N. Engl. J. Med.* 378: 2311–2320.

22. Cirino, A.L. and Ho, C. (1993). Hypertrophic cardiomyopathy overview. In: *GeneReviews*® (ed. M.P. Adam, H.H. Ardinger, R.A. Pagon, et al.). Seattle, WA: University of Washington.

23. Centers for Disease and Prevention (2008). Update on overall prevalence of major birth defects – Atlanta, Georgia, 1978–2005. *MMWR Morb. Mortal. Wkly Rep.* 57: 1–5.

24. Feldkamp, M.L., Carey, J.C., Byrne, J.L.B. et al. (2017). Etiology and clinical presentation of birth defects: population based study. *BMJ* 357: j2249.

Chapter 6

25. Gonzaga-Jauregui, C. and Lupski, J.R. (2021). *Genomics of Rare Diseases: Understanding Disease Genetics Using Genomic Approaches*. San Diego, CA: (Academic Press).

26. Bennett, R.L., French, K.S., Resta, R.G., and Doyle, D.L. (2008). Standardized human pedigree nomenclature: update and assessment of the recommendations of the National Society of Genetic Counselors. *J. Genet. Couns.* 17: 424–433.

27. Galvan-Femenia, I., Barcelo-Vidal, C., Sumoy, L. et al. (2021). A likelihood ratio approach for identifying three-quarter siblings in genetic databases. *Heredity (Edinb)* 126: 537–547.

28. White, M.B., Leppert, M., Nielsen, D. et al. (1991). A de novo cystic fibrosis mutation: CGA (Arg) to TGA (stop) at codon 851 of the CFTR gene. *Genomics* 11: 778–779.

29. Saranjam, H., Chopra, S.S., Levy, H. et al. (2013). A germline or de novo mutation in two families with Gaucher disease: implications for recessive disorders. *Eur. J. Hum. Genet.* 21: 115–117.

30. Ong, T., Marshall, S.G., Karczeski, B.A. et al. (1993). Cystic fibrosis and congenital absence of the vas deferens. In: *GeneReviews®* (ed. M.P. Adam, H.H. Ardinger, R.A. Pagon, et al.). Seattle, WA: University of Washington.

31. Stevenson, R.E., Allanson, J.G., Everman, D.B., and Solomon, B.D. (2016). *Human Malformations and Related Anomalies*. New York: Oxford University Press.

32. Alkuraya, F.S. (2012). Discovery of rare homozygous mutations from studies of consanguineous pedigrees. *Curr. Protoc. Hum. Genet.* 6 (Unit6): 12.

33. Solomon, B.D. and Muenke, M. (2012). When to suspect a genetic syndrome. *Am. Fam. Physician* 86: 826–833.

34. Bhinder, M.A., Sadia, H., Mahmood, N. et al. (2019). Consanguinity: a blessing or menace at population level? *Ann. Hum. Genet.* 83: 214–219.

35. Lapunzina, P. and Monk, D. (2011). The consequences of uniparental disomy and copy number neutral loss-of-heterozygosity during human development and cancer. *Biol. Cell.* 103: 303–317.

36. Soellner, L., Begemann, M., Mackay, D.J. et al. (2017). Recent advances in imprinting disorders. *Clin. Genet.* 91: 3–13.

37. Zhang, K., Astigarraga, I., Bryceson, Y. et al. (1993). Familial hemophagocytic lympho-histiocytosis. In: *GeneReviews®* (ed. M.P. Adam, H.H. Ardinger, R.A. Pagon, et al.). Seattle, WA: University of Washington.

38. National Cancer Institute Dictionaries. https://www.cancer.gov/publications/dictionaries/genetics-dictionary/def/phenocopy (accessed 26 July 21).

39. Yamamoto, F., Clausen, H., White, T. et al. (1990). Molecular genetic basis of the histo-blood group ABO system. *Nature* 345: 229–233.

40. Richards, S., Aziz, N., Bale, S. et al. (2015). Standards and guidelines for the interpretation of sequence variants: a joint consensus recommendation of the American College of Medical Genetics and Genomics and the Association for Molecular Pathology. *Genet. Med.* 17: 405–424.

41. Tsai, G.J., Ranola, J.M.O., Smith, C. et al. (2019). Outcomes of 92 patient-driven family studies for reclassification of variants of uncertain significance. *Genet. Med.* 21: 1435–1442.

42. Torkamani, A., Wineinger, N.E., and Topol, E.J. (2018). The personal and clinical utility of polygenic risk scores. *Nat. Rev. Genet.* 19: 581–590.

43. Sugrue, L.P. and Desikan, R.S. (2019). What are polygenic scores and why are they important? *JAMA* 321: 1820–1821.
44. Ogino, S. and Wilson, R.B. (2004). Bayesian analysis and risk assessment in genetic counseling and testing. *J. Mol. Diagn.* 6: 1–9.
45. Schild, R.L., Hunt, G.H., Moore, J. et al. (1996). Antenatal sonographic diagnosis of thanatophoric dysplasia: a report of three cases and a review of the literature with special emphasis on the differential diagnosis. *Ultrasound Obstet. Gynecol.* 8: 62–67.
46. French, T. and Savarirayan, R. (1993). Thanatophoric dysplasia. In: *GeneReviews*® (ed. M.P. Adam, H.H. Ardinger, R.A. Pagon, et al.). Seattle, WA: University of Washington.
47. Gyato, K., Wray, J., Huang, Z.J. et al. (2004). Metabolic and neuropsychological phenotype in women heterozygous for ornithine transcarbamylase deficiency. *Ann. Neurol.* 55: 80–86.
48. Lichter-Konecki, U., Caldovic, L., Morizono, H., and Simpson, K. (1993). Ornithine transcarbamylase deficiency. In: *GeneReviews*® (ed. M.P. Adam, H.H. Ardinger, R.A. Pagon, et al.). Seattle, WA: University of Washington.
49. Kalia, S.S., Adelman, K., Bale, S.J. et al. (2017). Recommendations for reporting of secondary findings in clinical exome and genome sequencing, 2016 update (ACMG SF v2.0): a policy statement of the American College of Medical Genetics and Genomics. *Genet. Med.* 19: 249–255.

Chapter 6

Index

Notes:

1. Additional terms for medical conditions can be found in databases, such as at: https://www.omim.org/.

2. In general, the names of medical conditions may be written and punctuated in different ways. For this book, with some exceptions based on common usage, we have tried to consistently capitalize the first word of specific condition names (if not already capitalized due to the use of an eponym).

Medical Genetics and Genomics: Questions for Board Review, First Edition. Benjamin D. Solomon.
© 2023 John Wiley & Sons Ltd. Published 2023 by John Wiley & Sons Ltd.

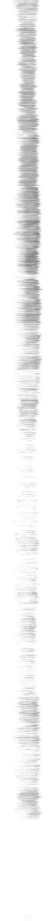